American Dietetic Association Guide to Eating Right When You Have Diabetes

American Dietetic Association Guide to Eating Right When You Have Diabetes

Maggie Powers, M.S., R.D., C.D.E.

JOHN WILEY & SONS, INC.

Published by John Wiley & Sons, Inc., Hoboken, New Jersey
Published simultaneously in Canada

Design and production by Navta Associates, Inc.

For general information about our other products and services, please contact our Customer Care Department within the United States at (800) 762-2974, outside the United States at (317) 572-3993 or fax (317) 572-4002.

Wiley also publishes its books in a variety of electronic formats. Some content that appears in print may not be available in electronic books. For more information about Wiley products, visit our web site at www.wiley.com.

Library of Congress Cataloging-in-Publication Data:

Powers, Maggie.
   American Dietetic Association guide to eating right when you have
diabetes / Maggie Powers.
      p. ; cm.
   Includes bibliographical references and index.
   ISBN 0-471-44222-4 (paper : alk. paper)
   1. Diabetes—Diet therapy.
      [DNLM: 1. Diabetic Diet—Popular Works. 2. Diabetes Mellitus, Non-Insulin-
Dependent—prevention & control—Popular Workds. 3. Dietary Carbohydrates—
Popular Works. 4. Dietary Supplements—Popular Works. WK 818 P888a 2003]
   I. Title: Guide to eating right when you have diabetes. II. American Dietetic
Association. III. Title.
   RC662 .P688 2003
   616.4'620654—dc21   2002014018

Printed in the United States of America

   4 5 6 7 8 9 10

This book is dedicated to my mother—Peg Nickels— who has type 2 diabetes and right before her eightieth birthday switched from diabetes pills to four injections of insulin a day. Her spirit, kindness, and take-it-as-it-comes attitude are truly an inspiration.

Contents

Acknowledgments

Thank you to all who were involved in the many aspects of writing this book, including:

- Those who may not even know they contributed—the many people who live with diabetes every day, the health professionals who provide diabetes care and influence me by the things they do every day, and the lady on the plane whose mom has diabetes—all touch me many ways.

- Those at the American Dietetic Association who contributed to the initiation and development of this book, especially Laura Brown, Diana Faulhaber, Anne Coghill, June Zaragoza, and Deborah McBride.

- Those at John Wiley & Sons, Inc., for their commitment to publishing this book, along with their insights, and vision for making it a terrific resource to all who live with diabetes, especially Elizabeth Zack, Linda Schonberg, and Lisa Burstiner.

- Kimberly Rinderknecht and Melissa Fredricks, who designed the menus and did the nutrient analysis; Ellen Tani, who did statistical research; and Sue Narayan, who provided editorial reviews.

- Expert reviewers Connie Crawley and Sandy Gillespie for their insightful comments and thoughtful reviews that helped shape and sharpen each chapter.

- Special friends and colleagues Mary Austin and Karmeen Kulkarni for being there with support and reviewer expertise through each phase of this exciting adventure.

- Many colleagues and friends who inspire me to pursue quality and balance in my life.

- And, of course, my husband and children, who accept me delving into exciting projects, give me encouragement, listen, and help me find better ways to explain "things." A special thank you to Mike, Jessica, Colin, and Martin.

Introduction

"What can I eat?" If you have diabetes you probably think about this question a lot. In fact, it is the most common question that people with diabetes ask. This book answers this question and many others related to food and diabetes. It is your daily guide in caring for your diabetes.

The theme of this book is that every person with diabetes is an individual first who happens to have diabetes. This means that the foods you like to eat and the schedule you like to keep are the foundation of your diabetes care plan. Throughout the book you will be guided in making decisions that fit your particular situation. The book will encourage you to set goals that are meaningful to you and give you confidence in your choices.

You gain confidence and control of your daily decisions when you know how food affects your blood glucose. Each section of the book will help you know more about how food affects your blood glucose.

Part One, "Understanding Diabetes," talks about setting goals that are important and meaningful to you, what diabetes is, and how the different types are treated. It moves you through the beginning discussions about what foods you like to eat, different types of food plans, and establishing your own food plan. It includes a whole week of menus to get you started or to give you a break from planning meals.

Part Two, "Key Aspects of Diabetes Care," explains why blood glucose monitoring, being active, losing weight, and preventing low blood glucose levels are usually the important initial subjects of discussion when someone has diabetes. These chapters give you information so you can personalize diabetes and food decisions to fit your needs.

Part Three, "Knowing What's in Food," is an interesting section about why we need a variety of food and how different amounts of food affect our blood glucose levels and our nutrient needs. Controlling blood fats and blood pressure are highlighted in this section because they are an important part of diabetes care and are affected by the food you eat.

Part Four, "Planning Your Meals," takes you to more specific steps in choosing your foods. The traditional Exchange System is explained, as is the widely used Carbohydrate Counting method of meal planning. Even if you opt to use one of the other food planning guidelines described in the first section, these two chapters will give you insight into making food choices and planning meals.

Part Five, "Tips for Choosing Foods," adds a little bit extra about everyday situations that affect your food choices. From how to read a food label to how to adjust your food plan when you eat late, you will find lots of tips to boost your everyday comfort in choosing foods.

The appendixes add further tips and guides for finding a dietitian and making food decisions. This book is packed with a lot of information and details about diabetes and food and is written with the authority of the American Dietetic Association, so there's a lot of excellent information about how to manage your diabetes effectively through the right food choices. But you will also need a diabetes care team. A dietitian is a key member of your team who has food and nutrient information readily available, can help you find your personal diabetes balance with the food you like to eat, and will guide and support you in achieving your diabetes goals.

May you find great comfort in making food choices and success in achieving your goals.

PART ONE

Understanding Diabetes

CHAPTER 1

Planning for Success

The most challenging aspect of diabetes care for many people is making food choices. This includes knowing what to eat, when to eat, how much to eat, and how to prepare food. It also includes knowing how to adjust food intake when blood glucose is high or low, when physically active, when traveling, when sick, and during other situations. This book will be your guide in making these types of decisions—it will help you plan for success.

This book will serve as your map for making food choices. It is like the maps we use for driving, especially when going to new or unfamiliar places. After you have driven to a place several times it gets easier, and eventually becomes second nature. This is just like caring for your diabetes and making food choices. Some parts of diabetes care can easily become habits while other parts may require a road map, specific directions, and even support in understanding the directions.

This book puts you in the driver's seat in that it helps to map out your diabetes food plan and provides directions for achieving your diabetes and nutritional goals. This chapter will help you:

- Identify your diabetes goals
- Know the purpose of a diabetes food plan
- Know who should be part of your diabetes care team

DIABETES GOALS

Your individual diabetes goals determine the direction of your overall diabetes care. Some examples of specific goals of diabetes care that you might have include wanting to:

- Feel better
- Have more energy
- See better without blurred vision
- Sleep better—not get up so many times at night to go to the bathroom
- Have a better memory
- Think more clearly
- Experience fewer infections
- Have good sexual function
- Have a strong heart and healthy kidneys
- Prevent diabetes complications

Taking care of your diabetes takes time and effort. Think about what would help make it worthwhile for you. Would reaching one of these goals help? Perhaps there is another goal that is more important to you. Think about these diabetes goals, and then talk to your diabetes care team about them in the order of their importance to you.

YOUR DIABETES FOOD PLAN

Your diabetes food plan is an important part of caring for your diabetes. The purpose of a diabetes food plan is to help you:

- Be in control of your:
  Blood glucose

Blood fats

Blood pressure
- Prevent, delay, or treat complications
- Improve your health

Obviously, your food plan is a critical part of your diabetes care. Your food plan, however, does not need to be a strict, rigid diet. Rather, you should be able to continue to enjoy eating foods you like and are accustomed to eating. You may need to modify your usual eating pattern to achieve your diabetes goals. Small changes can be made one at a time so you can become comfortable with them and then move on to additional changes, if necessary.

YOUR DIABETES CARE TEAM

You do not need to manage your diabetes by yourself, nor should you. You are in charge of your diabetes care and have a lot to think about and manage. Your diabetes care team will help you learn what you need to know about diabetes and help you make any changes you want to make.

Because a food plan is an essential part of your diabetes care, an expert in food and nutrition should be on your diabetes team. Registered dietitians can help you feel comfortable with the many food and diabetes decisions you are faced with every day. See the following box for the top five reasons to see a dietitian. Appendix A lists resources for finding a dietitian near you and questions you might want to ask.

Who should be on your diabetes care team?

- A doctor or nurse practitioner who will be your primary health care provider. He or she will oversee your health care and will write prescriptions and order tests. You may also regularly or occasionally see a diabetes specialist (endocrinologist or diabetologist) for an assessment of your diabetes treatment plan. If you do, your specialist will consult with your primary health care provider about your diabetes treatment.

Top Five Reasons to Talk to a Dietitian

1. You're new to diabetes and don't know what to eat.
2. You've had diabetes awhile but need to get back on track.
3. You want help in deciding how to eat your favorite foods.
4. Your schedule makes it difficult to eat well.
5. You want to feel better and improve your diabetes control.

Also, see your dietitian at least two to four times a year for a review of your food plan and blood glucose records, and to learn about any new updates.

- A Registered Dietitian (RD) who will help you understand all about the relationship between food and diabetes. She will help you select what to eat, understand how food affects your blood glucose blood fat and blood pressure levels, and help you evaluate your diabetes care plan from a food perspective. Your dietitian will review your daily blood glucose monitoring records, your medications, your activity, and your food intake. Let her know what your concerns are, what specific help you want, and what motivates you. She will then discuss ways to improve your diabetes control so you can choose which steps you want to take.
- A certified diabetes educator (CDE), who may be the dietitian you see (many dietitians are also CDEs) or another health professional (often a nurse or a pharmacist). The CDE will help you with other aspects of diabetes care such as understanding the complications of diabetes, selecting a glucose meter, knowing how to check your feet every day, and injecting insulin.
- Other health care professionals may be part of your regular or yearly diabetes care including a physical or occupational therapist, psychotherapist, social worker, podiatrist, and ophthalmologist or optometrist. There may be others, depending on your health needs and goals.

In addition to your diabetes team, there are other resources to help you in all areas of diabetes care. See appendix A for helpful resources. You may receive advice from your family, friends, and even strangers about diabetes. This advice may be valuable, but be sure it is best for you and your diabetes, because what works for one person is not always recommended for someone else. Because of this very reason, this book gives a variety of examples and choices for different situations so that you and your diabetes care team can select the best path for you.

CHAPTER 2

Understanding Diabetes

There is a lot to know about diabetes. This chapter helps you understand what diabetes is and why your food plan is an important part of your diabetes care. This chapter will:

- Review what diabetes is and what insulin does
- Give an overview of diabetes medicines
- Describe blood glucose values used to evaluate diabetes control

WHAT IS DIABETES?

Diabetes is a medical condition caused by a lack or inefficient use of insulin. Either your body produces no insulin, or it is unable to use the insulin it makes. Fortunately, your diabetes care team can help you understand how your body does or does not make insulin, and determine the best way to care for your diabetes. Diabetes care focuses on how to balance what you eat with the amount of insulin you have or take. When your insulin is balanced right for you, your body functions smoothly and you can efficiently process the food you eat.

A typical sign of diabetes is high blood glucose. When you eat, your food gets digested and some of it ends up as glucose in your blood. That glucose is very important. It gets carried throughout your body and is used as energy or stored for future use. Some of your body's cells can't use glucose unless there is insulin. Insulin is like the key that unlocks the door to your cells so that glucose can get into the cells.

Some say that "insulin opens the gates" or that "insulin is like the key that starts a car" or "the match that starts a fire." If you don't have enough insulin or can't use your insulin efficiently, you can't unlock the doors, can't open the gates, can't start the car, or can't start the fire.

Without the right amount of insulin, you can become tired and dehydrated, your eyesight may be blurry, and you may have sores that don't heal. This can change with a diabetes care plan that corrects the situation and gives you the right balance of food, activity, and insulin.

The pancreas (a body organ like the kidneys and liver, located on the left side of your body behind your lower ribs) makes insulin—a little bit all day long, and then in two bursts after a meal, when there is a rise in blood glucose. Insulin also controls other functions in your body related to the food you eat and these are listed in the following box.

After you eat, insulin:
- Lets glucose into the cells to be used for energy or stored for later energy
- Lets fat into the cells to be used for energy or stored for later energy
- Lets protein be used to repair cells, organs, and muscle

If insulin is not available or cannot do its work:
- Glucose stays in the blood
- Fat stays in the blood
- Protein is not used to repair cells, organs, and muscle

THE FOCUS OF DIABETES CARE

Diabetes care focuses on controlling a person's blood glucose level with an individualized food plan, an activity plan, and, if needed, medication. The care, treatment, or management of diabetes is often referred to as "controlling blood glucose levels." Control means keeping your blood glucose levels not too high and not too low. This book will help you learn how to make decisions so you can "control" your blood glucose.

The primary indicators of blood glucose control are your blood glucose checks and A1C values. When these values move toward, or are near, the values of a person without diabetes then you will have less risk of developing complications of diabetes (such as heart disease, eye problems, and kidney disease). That is why so much emphasis is put on blood glucose control—because that is how you prevent complications and can achieve a variety of goals, such as those listed in chapter 1 (see page 8).

To think about the balance you need to achieve blood glucose control, think about a three-legged stool. One leg of the stool is insulin, and the other two are food and activity. If one leg is too short, there is an imbalance. The focus of diabetes care is to find the right balance of the food you eat, your physical activity levels, and the insulin you make or take. Who sits on the stool also affects the balance; this is your diabetes and you need to find the balance that is right for you. When your blood glucose is under control, then you have the right balance.

THE DIFFERENT TYPES OF DIABETES

In North America alone, almost 20 million people—over 17 million in the United States and over 2 million in Canada—have diabetes. More than 6 million do not know they have it and therefore cannot take the steps to care for it. Caring for diabetes means treating the elevated blood glucose levels to prevent the complications that are associated with uncontrolled diabetes. To help understand your diabetes needs, let's discuss the three types of diabetes: type 1, type 2, and gestational diabetes.

Type 1 Diabetes

Approximately 500,000 to 1 million people in North America have type 1 diabetes, some as young as a couple of months old and adults who have lived over 50 years with diabetes. Although typically diagnosed before the age of 30 years, type 1 diabetes can be diagnosed in older individuals. Every person with type 1 diabetes needs to take insulin every day since they make no insulin, or very, very little. The treatment plan always includes insulin and a food plan.

Insulin is a protein and, in its current form, must be given by injection or by an insulin pump. Research is currently being conducted on how to deliver insulin in other ways, including as an oral aerosol spray and an inhaled insulin powder.

You and your diabetes care team will design an insulin plan (sometimes called insulin regimen) that you will follow each day. It will tell you what type of insulin to take at different times of the day. It can consist of two shots of insulin each day, three to four shots a day, or an insulin pump that delivers the insulin in precise amounts throughout the day.

Your insulin plan will affect the timing of your meals and how much food should be eaten. For this reason, your insulin regimen should match your typical eating pattern. Your diabetes team will help you find the regimen that most easily fits your schedule, and will help you change it when your schedule or eating habits change.

In general, there are two types of insulin plans for those with type 1 diabetes. They are described here with comments about the food choices for each one.

- Two shots a day, each with usually two kinds of insulin. You can mix your insulin yourself, or use a premixed insulin. If you use a premixed insulin then you need to be very consistent with the timing and amount of food you eat.
- Three or four shots a day or an insulin pump. With this regimen, you will be adjusting the amount of rapid- or short-acting insulin before each meal. This gives you flexibility in the timing of when you eat and how much you eat. The insulin plan can be adjusted to fit your typical eating pattern and various foods you may consume. For example, if you want to eat more for lunch, you can take a predetermined extra amount of insulin to cover the expected additional rise in your blood glucose. How to do this is explained in chapter 14.

The table opposite lists the characteristics of the different types of insulin including when the insulin begins to work, is working hardest, and when it stops working.

The illustrations in Figures 1 through 3 show how insulin works based on its characteristics.

If you take insulin, you can draw your insulin's action in the blank area of Figure 4. Do this to help better understand how your insulin works and how food relates to your insulin.

Your diabetes care team will help you with more specifics, but several key points about food and insulin are:

- Take a rapid-acting insulin right before you eat because it starts to work almost immediately. Some say, "Dose and eat."
- Take a short-acting insulin 30 minutes before you eat.
- Intermediate-acting insulin peaks 4–10 hours after you take it. If you often have low blood glucose episodes about that time, you can make a change in your food, activity, or insulin so that doesn't happen.

The long-acting insulin typically has no peak action, yet some find it does. If you are having a low blood glucose episode that is difficult to explain, consider this.

Insulin Action Times

Bolus Insulin	Begins to Work	Working Hardest	Stops Working Effectively
Rapid-acting			
Lispro (Humalog®)	5–15 minutes	30–75 minutes	2–4 hours
Aspart (Novolog®)	5–15 minutes	1–2 hours	3–6 hours
Short-acting			
Regular	30–45 minutes	2–3 hours	4–8 hours

Background Insulin			
Intermediate-acting			
NPH	2–4 hours	4–8 hours	10–16 hours
Lente	2–4 hours	4–8 hours	10–16 hours
Prolonged intermediate-acting			
Ultralente	3–5 hours	8–12 hours	18–20 hours
Long-acting			
Glargine (Lantus®)	4–8 hours	No peak	24 hours

Premixed Insulin			
Background/Bolus		*Early peak–Late peak*	
75/25 with Lis or 70/30 with Asp	5–15 minutes	1–12 hours	About 18 hours
70/30 with Reg or 50/50	30–60 minutes	2–12 hours	About 18 hours

Source: Insulin BASICS Clinical Guidelines. International Diabetes Center, Minneapolis, MN, 2002. Used with permission.

Some people will take several insulins at a time or throughout the day. The rapid- and short-acting insulins are typically taken before meals. They are called bolus insulins because they are used to cover a rise in blood glucose from a meal. The intermediate- and long-acting insulins are used to provide insulin coverage when the rapid- and short-acting insulins are not working and are often called background or basal insulins.

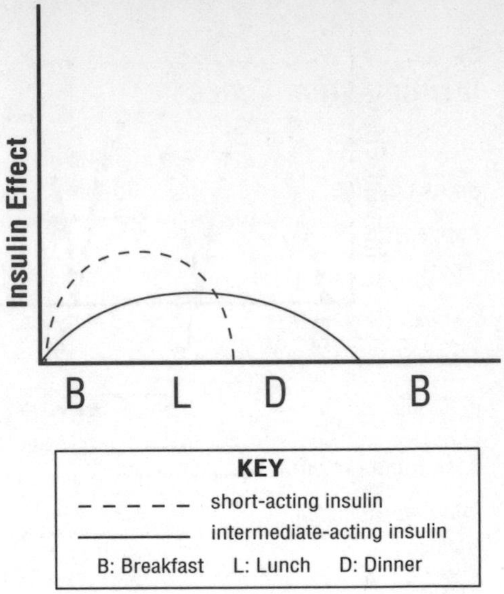

Figure 1 Mixed dose of short-acting and intermediate-acting insulins at breakfast.* This could be a mixed dose of rapid-acting and intermediate-acting insulins. You may also take an injection of intermediate-acting insulin at bedtime.

Insulin Effect

B   L   D   B

KEY

– – – – – short-acting insulin

———— intermediate-acting insulin

B: Breakfast   L: Lunch   D: Dinner

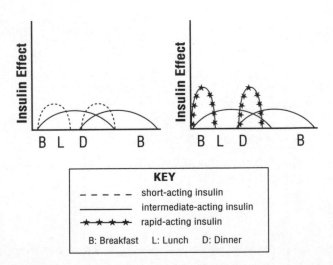

KEY

– – – – – short-acting insulin

———— intermediate-acting insulin

★★★★★ rapid-acting insulin

B: Breakfast   L: Lunch   D: Dinner

Figure 2 Split mixed dose of two injections of insulin given before breakfast and dinner. The left drawing is short-acting with intermediate-acting insulin. The right drawing is rapid-acting with intermediate-acting.*

* You can mix short-acting insulin or rapid-acting insulin with intermediate-acting insulin in one insulin syringe or use a premixed insulin. Currently glargine cannot be mixed with other insulins.

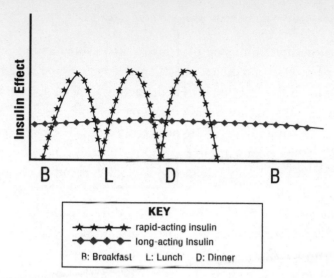

Figure 3 Four injections of insulin a day. An injection of rapid-acting before each meal and long-acting (glargine) either at bedtime or in the morning.

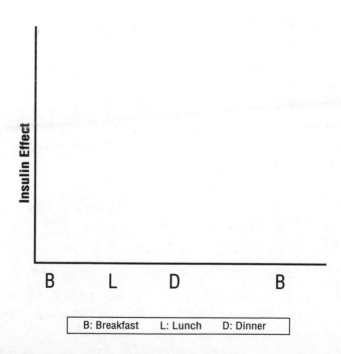

Figure 4 Draw your current insulin regimen here.

For example, someone may take a little short-acting insulin before breakfast and dinner but will need insulin to be available all day long, so they may mix the short-acting with an intermediate-acting insulin. Mixing means drawing up both insulins in one syringe so you only need one needle injection. There are specific guidelines for mixing insulins and some insulins cannot be mixed. Be sure to talk to your diabetes care team about your specific insulin guidelines.

One guideline that you may want to discuss is the variation in timing of injecting rapid- or short-acting insulin. Since the rapid-acting insulin starts its action so quickly and has a fairly short duration, it offers some flexibility in its use. It is especially helpful with children who have difficulty understanding the importance of eating a certain amount of food at a meal. The rapid-acting insulin dosage can be given after the meal to match the amount of food that was consumed. Another variation can be that if the blood glucose level before a meal is a little higher than usual, the rapid- or short-acting insulin can be taken earlier than usually recommended. Again, discuss these types of guidelines with your diabetes care team because everyone's situation is a little bit different.

For those who don't want to mix their own insulin, there are premixed insulins. There are premixes of background and bolus insulins:

> **Know Your Insulin**
>
> If you take insulin, find the insulin regimen that most closely matches your insulin regimen. Are you eating when the insulin's action is the greatest? Is there an insulin regimen that fits your eating style better? Do not change it yourself, but discuss it with your primary care provider.

- 75/25 = 75% intermediate- + 25% rapid-acting (Lispro)
- 70/30A = 70% intermediate- + 30% rapid-acting (Aspart)
- 70/30R = 70% intermediate- + 30% short-acting (regular)
- 50/50 = 50% intermediate- + 50% short-acting

and a pre-mix of intermediate- and rapid-acting insulins.

These insulin mixtures are quite popular, but do have some limitations. They do not allow one to adjust the rapid- or short-acting insulin based on what they are going to eat. The tradeoff is that one can easily use a mixed insulin, and for many adjusting the rapid- or short-acting insulin is not necessary.

Type 2 Diabetes

Some feel that type 2 diabetes is a less serious form of diabetes and that "just a touch of sugar" won't do any harm. Don't believe it; all diabetes is serious. According to the Centers for Disease Control and Prevention, diabetes is the seventh leading cause of death and a major contributor to the development of heart disease, stroke, blindness, high blood pressure, kidney disease, and amputations.

Almost 16 million people have type 2 diabetes in the United States; that is, over 90% of all people with diabetes have type 2 diabetes. Type 2 diabetes used to be called adult-onset diabetes because it was usually diagnosed in older adults. Today many young children are developing type 2 diabetes because they are inactive and overweight. Just like the adults with type 2, they do not make enough insulin, or they cannot use the insulin they make properly. The primary treatment of anyone with type 2 diabetes is a healthy food plan and regular physical activity.

The treatment plan may also include weight loss strategies because 80–90% of those with type 2 diabetes are overweight. The prevalence of type 2 diabetes has tripled in the last 30 years, and much of the increase is due to a rise in obesity. Small amounts of weight loss can dramatically improve blood glucose control, so losses of 10 to 20 pounds in adults are often suggested. Children may or may not need to lose weight because they are still growing. If you are not overweight, or choose to maintain your current weight, a food plan is still a necessary part of your diabetes care.

Two situations are common in persons with type 2 diabetes:

- *Insulin resistance* is when your body cannot use all of the insulin it produces. In fact, many make high amounts of insulin but the body resists using it. Losing some weight and being more active allows the body to use more easily the insulin it makes. New diabetes medicines also can help reduce insulin resistance.
- *Insulin deficiency* is when your pancreas does not make enough insulin. This often happens after years of insulin resistance and your pancreas is worn out from years of making high amounts of insulin and now is not able to produce much insulin. Eating smaller meals through out the day, rather than eating one or two large meals, may help you achieve blood glucose control. There are also diabetes medicines that can either help your pancreas make more insulin or help your body better use the insulin it makes.

Type 2 diabetes is a progressive disease, which means that if you have it for a long time, you will usually progress from needing just food and activity plans for treatment to adding a diabetes pill (or pills) and then insulin. About half of all people with type 2 diabetes take insulin. Your goal? Be aggressive with your food and activity plans during all stages of diabetes treatment, even the early stages. This may help you achieve blood glucose control that will hopefully delay the progression of your diabetes.

There are a variety of diabetes pills available that:

- Help the pancreas make more insulin
- Help the body use insulin better
- Prevent the liver from making more glucose
- Slow the digestion of some carbohydrates

These pills can be taken with each other or with insulin. See the following table for a list of the different types of diabetes pills. Discuss when to take your diabetes pills with your diabetes care team and know if there are any specific steps you need to follow. For example, Prandin should be taken right before you start eating, or ideally within 15 minutes before a meal, and not taken if a meal is skipped; Glyset and Precose should be taken with the first bite of food.

ORAL AGENTS

Generic Name	Trade Name	Common Starting Dose	Maximum Daily Dose	Schedule for Taking
Sulfonylureas: *Stimulate the pancreas to release more insulin.*				
Glyburide	Diabeta	1.25–5.0 mg	20 mg	1–2 times daily with meals
	Micronase	1.25–5.0 mg	20 mg	1–2 times daily with meals
	Glynase	1.5–3.0 mg	12 mg	1–2 times daily with meals
Glipizide	Glucotrol	5.0 mg	40 mg	1–2 times daily ½ hr. before meals
	Glucotrol XL (extended release)	2.5 – 5.0 mg	20 mg	1–2 times daily with meals
Glimepiride	Amaryl	1.0–2.0 mg	8.0 mg	1 time daily with meal
Biguanides: *Decrease glucose released by liver and make cells more sensitive to insulin.*				
Metformin	Glucophage	500–1,000 mg	2,550 mg	1–3 times daily with meals
Metformin	Glucophage XR	500 mg	2,000 mg	1 time daily with evening meal
Sulfonylurea/Biguanide				
Glyburide and Metformin HCl	Glucovance	1.25 mg/ 250 mg or 2.5 mg/ 500 mg	20 mg/ 2,000 mg	1–2 times daily with meals
Meglitinides: *Stimulate the pancreas to release a burst of insulin.*				
Repaglinide	Prandin	0.5–1.0 mg	16 mg	2–4 times daily with meals
D-phenylalanine Derivatives: *Stimulate the pancreas to release a burst of insulin.*				
Nateglinide	Starlix	120 mg	480 mg	2–4 times daily with meals

(continued)

ORAL AGENTS *(continued)*

Generic Name	Trade Name	Common Starting Dose	Maximum Daily Dose	Schedule for Taking
Thiazolidinediones: *Make cells more sensitive to insulin and decrease glucose released by liver.*				
Rosiglitazone	Avandia	4.0 mg	8.0 mg	1–2 times daily
Pioglitazone	Actos	15–30 mg	45 mg	1 time daily
Alpha Glucosidase Inhibitors: *Slow the absorption of carbohydrates.*				
Acarbose	Precose	25 mg	300 mg	3 times daily with meals
Miglitol	Glyset	25 mg	300 mg	3 times daily with meals

New medications and formulations are approved by the Food and Drug Administration on an ongoing basis. Ask your health care provider for the latest information.

Source: Insulin BASICS Clinical Guidelines. International Diabetes Center, Minneapolis, MN, 2002. Used with permission.

Diabetes medications only supplement your food and activity plans. You must continue to follow your food and activity plans, and may need to be more precise with the timing and amount of food you eat once you start taking a diabetes medicine.

Gestational Diabetes

Gestational diabetes mellitus (GDM) is typically diagnosed during the twenty-fourth to twenty-eighth week of pregnancy. GDM happens when the pancreas is unable to produce the extra insulin that is needed during the last part of a pregnancy. Treatment always begins with a food plan and diligent monitoring of blood glucose levels throughout the day. The amount of carbohydrate at meals and snacks is carefully monitored and distributed based on blood glucose results. One should never stop eating in order to improve blood glucose levels, because the mother and the growing infant need food.

It is critical that the mother's blood glucose stay within approved guidelines, for the health and safety of both the mother and infant. The American Diabetes Association recommends starting a diabetes medication if a food plan alone cannot keep the fasting blood glucose to 95 mg/dl or below, or the one-hour-after-meal blood glucose to 140 mg/dl or below. (These values are for whole blood; plasma values are as follows: below 105 mg/dl for fasting and below 155 mg/dl for one-hour-after-meal.) Typically insulin is started, but new research shows that one of the diabetes pills (Glyburide) does not cross the placenta, and may be acceptable to use with GDM.

After the infant is delivered, blood glucose levels return to normal. However, women who have had GDM are at an increased risk for later developing type 2 diabetes. About half the women who have GDM will develop type 2 diabetes within 15 to 20 years. For that reason, it is highly recommended that someone who had GDM maintain a healthy weight and be physically active to delay or prevent the onset of type 2 diabetes. A registered dietitian, who can help you with a food plan during your pregnancy, can be of great assistance after your pregnancy. Also, see appendix B on preventing diabetes.

BLOOD GLUCOSE CHECKS

A blood glucose check is a convenient way to know more about the food you eat. Blood glucose checks will tell you what your blood glucose level is at a particular time. That's why it is more appropriate to call it a "check" rather than a "test." You are checking to see what the effects of your food, activity, and insulin are at that particular time. Most importantly, they help you establish and evaluate your food plan. You can perform this simple check almost anywhere—at home, at work or school, in the car, or in a restaurant.

If you have never done a blood glucose check, it is a fairly simple procedure. You use a very small drop of your blood with a small glucose-measuring meter and will quickly get a number—your blood glucose value. A variety of glucose meters about the size of a deck of cards, or smaller, are available. They offer different features that may make one more suitable for you than another. To choose the right meter, consider the size of meter, size of drop of blood needed, and how long the check takes to do. There is a meter that measures glucose collected through the skin and does not require a drop of blood. More meters of this type are being developed to make blood glucose checks easier and more comfortable.

The results of your blood glucose checks are always feedback giving you information to use in making decisions about your diabetes care. If your blood glucose is high, that gives you information; if it is low, that also gives you information. Take charge of your diabetes and learn how to do blood glucose checks, what your target blood glucose goals are, and how to use the results of your blood glucose checks to improve your blood glucose control. Chapter 6 will give you specific guidelines for reviewing your blood glucose checks.

BLOOD GLUCOSE GOALS

The American Diabetes Association sets goals for blood glucose levels for before meals and at bedtime as listed in the following table. These goals are "target goals" and given as a range of numbers. When your blood glucose levels are close to the target goals, you decrease your risk for developing complications of diabetes.

Average Blood Glucose and A1C Goals

	Plasma (mg/dl)*	Whole Blood (mg/dl)
Before meals	90–130	80–120
2 hours after a meal†	Less than 160	Less than 150
At bedtime	110–150	100–140
A1C	Two to four times a year—less than 7%	

*Most glucose meters give plasma values.
†Values are not listed in position statement.
Source: American Diabetes Association: "Position Statement: Standards of medical care for patients with diabetes mellitus." *Diabetes Care* 25(S1), 2002, S33–S49.

Discuss and establish your target goals with your diabetes care team based on what is best for you. Your target blood glucose goals will depend on a variety of factors, including what other medical conditions you have, your living situation, your desire and ability to make lifestyle changes, what diabetes medicine you take, and whether you can feel if your blood glucose is low.

There is much interest in the blood glucose check done two hours after a meal (also called postprandial blood glucose). For a long time, checking after meals wasn't even suggested by most diabetes doctors. Now, it is considered an important time to check because it tells you so much. It tells you if you are eating the right amount of carbohydrate for the amount of insulin you make or you take. Once you know this, you and your diabetes care team can discuss possible changes such as eating less carbohydrate at that meal, changing diabetes medication, or changing physical activity.

It is generally recommended that this check is done two hours after you start eating. A common goal is to be less than 160 mg/dl. For some, the two-hour goal may be higher, yet the American Association of Clinical Endocrinologists recommends that the goal should be less than 140 mg/dl. Your diabetes care team can help you evaluate your target goals for after meals.

Blood glucose goals are summarized in the previous table and are given as plasma and whole blood values. The drop of blood you check with your glucose meter is known as *whole blood*. Yet, most meters will convert this number to a *plasma value*. This is done because the blood drawn from your arm at your doctor's visits is tested for plasma glucose. Plasma is more concentrated so the plasma values will be about 10% higher than whole blood values. Check your meter so you know what result you are getting.

The blood glucose goals listed in the previous table are averages. Some of your results will be at the high range, or even higher, while other results will be at the lower range. The International Diabetes Center in Minneapolis, Minnesota, has found that when 50% or more of your glucose checks are within your target range, your A1C will usually be in the target range too. Their goals are similar to the ADA goals: before meals 70–140 mg/dl, two hours after meals less than 160 mg/dl, and before bedtime 100–140 mg/dl. Individualize your goals with your diabetes care team. The goals for pregnant women are usually set lower, and goals for young children and some older adults may be a little higher. The A1C value is explained in the following section.

THE A1C TEST

The A1C test provides information about the average amount of glucose that has been in your blood during the previous two to three months. This test is another way to see if you are reaching your blood glucose goals. It measures the amount of glucose attached to the hemoglobin molecule in the blood and is done two to four times a year. Other names for this test include: hemoglobin A1C, glyco-hemoglobin, glycosolated hemoglobin, and glycated hemoglobin. All mean glucose that is attached to hemoglobin.

The following table shows how the A1C test relates to the average blood glucose level. For example, if your A1C is 8% your *average* blood glucose level over the previous two to three months has been 180. Note that it represents an average. That means some of your blood glucose checks will be higher and some will be lower.

The A1C test is often done at a laboratory from blood drawn from your arm, or it can be done in a doctor's office using blood from a finger stick. There are several blood glucose meters that also do a test similar to the A1C— a fructosamine test. The fructosamine test measures the amount of glucose attached to protein over the previous two to three *weeks*.

Review Your Records

Take a yellow marker and highlight all of your blood glucose checks that are in your target range. If half of your checks are in your target range, you should be able to meet your A1C goal.

Average Blood Glucose Levels Represented by an A1C Value

A1C (%)*	Average Blood Glucose Level (mg/dl)*
5	90
6	120
7	150
8	180
9	210
10	240
11	270
12	300
13	330
14	360

*A1C value should be kept in nonshaded levels.

Thus it gives a quicker indication of average blood glucose levels than the A1C does, which may be helpful in assessing treatment changes. Although it is not widely used, this test can be done at home.

It is possible that your daily blood glucose checks will be fine, but your A1C (or fructosamine) will be high. You will need to figure out why there is a difference.

Several reasons why the A1C test may be higher than daily blood glucose levels would predict include that your glucose meter is not working correctly or that you're checking your blood glucose when it is in your target blood glucose range but you need to check it at other times of the day when it may be high. It is the latter reason that has drawn more attention to the after-meal blood glucose checks and the discussion about what the target goal should be. If your A1C is higher than expected, check more frequently two hours after you start eating. If this value is above your goal, then you may want to adjust what you are eating, your activity, or your diabetes medication. Chapter 6 will give you some examples of what can be done, but be sure to discuss this with your dietitian and diabetes team.

Occasionally someone's A1C may be lower than expected; this is when blood glucose checks are high and A1C level is low. The glucose meter needs to be checked to be sure it is working correctly. Also, this may be due to a low level of hemoglobin due to anemia or kidney disease. Your diabetes care team can help you figure out why this happened.

In a number of research studies, patients whose A1C values had been closest to the American Diabetes Association's recommended goal of 7% have developed fewer complications of diabetes. Every decrease in your A1C levels will reduce your risk. Even going from 9.7% to 9% or going from 8.5% to 7.6% will help you decrease your risk and is worthy of celebration. If your A1C is above 7%, talk to your diabetes care team. They can discuss changes in your treatment plan to help you keep your A1C below that level.

PART TWO

Starting Your Food Plan

CHAPTER 3

Keeping a Food Diary

A food plan is an essential part of diabetes care and blood glucose control. Keeping a food diary will help you (1) design a food plan that includes the foods you like to eat; (2) know how your body responds to certain quantities of food; and (3) review your blood glucose records and guide decisions about how to change your diabetes management to better control your blood glucose.

Keep a food diary especially if you are just starting or restarting a food plan, beginning or adjusting your diabetes medication, have poor blood glucose control, have a schedule change, or are on a weight loss plan. Keep a food diary for at least a week or two so you can determine the best food plan, activity plan, and medication, if needed.

This chapter will help you:

- Know how to keep track of what you eat
- Use a food diary

YOUR FOOD DIARY

Each of us has our own eating style based on our family traditions, the culture we live in, and our own personal food likes and dislikes.

A food diary is a personal record of your eating style. By keeping a food diary, you may observe patterns in your eating that you hadn't noticed before. It is helpful to capture how you truly eat so that your diabetes food plan reflects *your* eating style, and not an eating style that is not yours.

Keep your food diary handy or in a special place that makes it easier to keep track of what you eat close to the time you actually consume the food or drink. It can be very easy to forget what you have eaten.

You will use this information to help you determine whether any of your eating habits need to be changed in order to meet your diabetes nutrition goals. Once you have developed a food plan that works for you in helping you meet your nutrition goals, you may not need to keep such detailed records. You may want to record two to four days once a month, just to be sure you are following your food plan. Or you may decide to continue to keep all your diabetes records in a daily food diary.

A Sample Food Diary

The following is a sample one-day food diary.

Appendix D contains a blank food diary that you can fill out or copy, allowing you to record as many days as you like. If it is easier for you, use your daily planner, a notepad, or a personal digital assistant (PDA) to keep this information.

Getting Started

Write down everything you consume, even if it is a snack, taste, or "nibble." Some people are quite surprised at how many snacks or nibbles they have in a day. When you write things down, you really see your eating style. You can decide later whether you need to make any changes. If you do not write something down, you may forget to include it in your food plan. The basic information you should record is listed in the following sample food diary:

My Sample Food Diary

Date: Monday, October 6

Time	Blood Glucose/ Meds	Everything I Ate and Drank Today and How Much	
7:30 A.M.	122 Glucophage 500 mg	Cereal	1½ cup wheat flakes ¾ cup 1% milk
		Coffee	1 cup ½ packet low-calorie sweetener
10:00 A.M.		1 chocolate candy bar	1 oz size
12:30 P.M.	165	Sandwich	2 slices whole wheat bread 3 oz turkey 1 piece lettuce 1 slice tomato 2 Tablespoons reduced-fat mayonnaise
		1% milk	1 cup
2:30 P.M.	180	Apple	medium sized
6:00 P.M.	166 Glucophage 500 mg	Soda crackers	12
		Salad (lettuce, tomato)	1 cup
		Dressing, creamy low-fat	2 Tablespoons
		Potatoes, mashed	1 cup
		Gravy	¼ cup
		Chicken with skin, grilled	1 breast
		Green beans, frozen	1 cup
		Water	2 cups
10:00 P.M.	123		

Today's activity and notes:

After dinner walked 1 miles in about 30 minutes

The time you eat. Write down the times of your all your meals and all snacks.

What and how much you eat. This is often the hardest part to record in your food diary. Is that scoop of potatoes a half cup, a cup, or two cups? The only way to know for sure is to measure. Vague measurements such as those listed in the following table make it difficult to define how much you eat. Surprisingly, many people with diabetes never measure their food, yet it is important to know how much you are eating. Then a food plan can be designed that takes into account how much food you like to eat.

Avoid Vague Measurements

This Serving:	Could Mean:
1 large bowl of cereal	1 to 3 cups
1 glass of juice	½ cup to 2 cups
1 scoop of rice	⅓ to 1 cup

Measuring with standard measuring equipment is recommended. You can observe your measured serving sizes so you can learn to accurately eye-measure to make it easier to keep your food diary. Then periodically check your estimated portions to be sure they are the size you think they are.

Other information. Include the results of your blood glucose checks, and note your activity for the day. If you take a diabetes medicine, weigh yourself, or take your blood pressure and pulse; add that information in the bottom box.

Some people like to include information about how they are feeling when they eat, who they ate with, and where they ate. This is especially useful if you are on a weight-loss food plan.

The food diary is your first step in establishing your food plan. It will be interesting—and probably surprising—to find out exactly what you eat. The goal of a personal food plan is to stay as close to your own eating style as possible. Your food diary is important in helping design your food plan and in reviewing your blood glucose records.

CHAPTER 4

Designing Your Food Plan

This chapter will help you:

- Begin to design a diabetes food plan
- Know about different food plans

THE BASIC FOCUS

A diabetes food plan is basically a healthy, all-around eating plan that will help you meet your diabetes nutrition goals. It follows the eating guidelines recommended for Americans (see the sidebar), as well as eating guidelines from other countries. They emphasize:

- Eating a variety of foods
- Limiting high-sugar, high-salt, and high-fat foods
- Eating to maintain a healthy weight

These are the same nutrition principles that guide the development of a diabetes food plan.

USDA Dietary Guidelines—10 Steps for Your Health

Aim for Fitness
- Aim for a healthy weight.
- Be physically active each day.

Build a Healthy Base
- Let the Food Guide Pyramid guide your food choices.
- Eat a variety of grains daily, especially whole grains.
- Eat a variety of fruits and vegetables daily.
- Keep food safe to eat.

Choose Sensibly
- Choose a diet that is low in saturated fat and cholesterol and moderate in total fat.
- Choose beverages and foods that limit your intake of sugars.
- Choose and prepare foods with less salt.
- If you drink alcoholic beverages, do so in moderation.

Source: Dietary Guidelines for Americans, 5th edition. United States Department of Agriculture, United States Department of Health and Human Services, 2000.

DESIGNING YOUR DIABETES FOOD PLAN

Your diabetes food plan is usually based on the foods you like to eat and your preferred daily schedule, as well as your diabetes goals. Keeping a food diary as suggested in chapter 3 is a good place to start. Keep a food diary for a week, and then review it to understand your typical eating pattern. Your eating pattern will be the foundation for your diabetes food plan. You will establish (1) usual eating times and (2) how much food you will eat at each time.

Chapter 6 will help you use blood glucose records to evaluate your food plan and overall diabetes treatment. For now, begin designing your food plan with the two steps listed above.

ESTABLISHING MEAL AND SNACK TIMES

Select times for each meal and snack that will be convenient for you on most days. Most people with diabetes have some flexibility with meal times. For example, if you choose to eat dinner at 6:00 P.M., a range from 5:30 to 6:30 should not be a problem. The general guideline is that a half-hour difference either earlier or later than your scheduled time usually doesn't affect blood glucose control.

Meal timing is most important for those with either type 1 or type 2 diabetes who take one to two injections of insulin a day. This is because the insulin is working whether you eat or don't eat. If you eat late the insulin is working and can cause a low blood glucose episode.

Food in the Morning

It's true that breakfast is the most important meal of the day. It helps you think better, be more creative, have more energy, be more focused, and be ready to learn or do work. It also helps you feel less irritable in the morning. With all these benefits, how could you not want to eat breakfast? Specifically for those with diabetes, eating breakfast helps spread your food intake through out the day making it easier to control your blood glucose levels. And it can help prevent overeating later in the day.

Despite these advantages, there are people who do not like to eat breakfast and people who like to sleep through breakfast on their days off. You do not *have to* eat breakfast. However, having meals and snacks spread throughout the day is recommended and referred to as meal spacing. If you normally don't eat breakfast, you may want to consider:

- *Eating a very small breakfast*—One piece of toast and half a glass of milk, one piece of fruit, or a breakfast bar.
- *Eating a morning snack*—One piece of fruit, peanut butter on crackers, a container of yogurt, a low-fat granola bar, or a small bagel.

Meal Spacing

Meal spacing is especially helpful for those who have type 2 diabetes and don't take a diabetes medicine. Try to space your meals four to five hours apart. This helps your pancreas to produce adequate amounts of insulin after each meal without over challenging it at any one time. Or, if you take a diabetes medication, spacing allows your diabetes medication time to work. The goal is to have your blood glucose return to your target range by the time you eat your next meal.

Snacks

Snacks are often not necessary unless you are planning vigorous activity, are a growing child, or are pregnant. Snacks used to be included in most diabetes food plans. Those on insulin usually had an afternoon and evening snack, and everyone else had an evening snack. Today, that is not necessary and your food plan can be designed with or without snacks.

Some of the reasons you may want to include a snack are that you eat small meals, you need a snack before activity, it's a convenient time to eat fruit which you might not like at meals, or you just like a snack at a certain time. Reasons to avoid snacks include that extra food for snacks can mean weight gain or increases in blood glucose levels. Discuss your preferences with your dietitian so your food plan is individualized for you.

Your Meal Times

What time do you usually eat? Review your food diary from chapter 3 and summarize your usual meal and snack times here.

Meal 1	Time	_____
Meal 2	Time	_____
Meal 3	Time	_____
Snack(s)	Time	_____ _____ _____ _____

ESTABLISHING HOW MUCH FOOD TO EAT

The second consideration in diabetes meal planning is the amount of food you eat at your meals and snacks each day. The amounts need to be fairly consistent from day to day, especially when you start taking a diabetes medication. Your goal then is to establish a usual amount of food for each meal and snack you eat.

You need to eat an adequate amount of food to meet your nutritional needs, so don't try to starve yourself in order to lower your blood glucose levels. Choose the amount of food that feels comfortable to you at each meal and try to consistently eat that amount. If, for example, your breakfast meal has a similar type and amount of food from day to day, then your blood glucose response after each breakfast will be about the same everyday. You need to be especially consistent about your carbohydrate-containing foods like breads, cereals, pastas, fruits, vegetables, and milk.

To determine if you are eating a consistent amount of food each day, first review your food record and compare your breakfast meals, lunches, dinners, and snacks to each other. Do your lunches contain about the same amount of food from day to day? If you eat a whole sandwich one day and half a sandwich the next day, that is not really consistent unless you had something extra like a bowl of soup with your half sandwich.

There are different ways to keep your food intake consistent from day to day. Eating the same thing every day is one way. However, this defeats one of the basic principles of a healthy diet—eating a variety of foods—and it will undoubtedly become quite boring. There are a variety of food planning guides to help you become more familiar with food choices. They will help you gain confidence in your food decisions and to comfortably expand your food choices.

FOOD PLANNING GUIDES

Some people are fairly consistent with their food amounts and only need to be concerned about eating meals at regular times. Others will need more specifics to achieve the balance their diabetes requires. Your food planning guide will help you decide what to eat. When you approach a table with various foods, a huge buffet table, a restaurant menu, or even your own refrigerator, you need to make a decision about what and how much you will eat. Your food plan guide helps you assess the food choices you have and make a decision.

You may want to use one type of food plan for several months or a year, then switch to another plan so you can have variety in your food options and not become bored with any one method. Review them, and then discuss the one you like best with your dietitian.

This next section describes a variety of diabetes meal planning methods. Dietitians use all of these, as well as variations of these. You can review them here and select one to follow, or discuss them all with your dietitian. The goal of each method is to help you select about the same amount of food to eat from day to day to help you meet your diabetes and nutrition goals.

General Diabetes Food Guidelines

If you eat fairly consistently from day to day and do not take a diabetes medication, then you may just need to follow general food guidelines. These guidelines are based on your usual food choices. A sample food plan using general guidelines might look like this:

- *Breakfast.* Have cereal with milk. Vary the type of cereal. Have a piece of fresh fruit or a half cup of fruit or juice.
- *Lunch.* Have a sandwich. Choose whole grain breads when possible, and have vegetables like lettuce and tomatoes on the sandwich or on the side. Have a piece of fresh fruit, and drink a glass of low-fat milk.
- *Dinner.* Have a large portion of vegetables or a salad, about one cup of starchy food (pasta, potatoes, rice, corn, or peas), and a piece of meat, fish, or poultry about the size of the palm of your hand. Enjoy fruit for dessert.

Actual portion sizes will vary depending on each person's calorie needs. For example, someone may need two sandwiches at lunch, and double the amount of starchy food at dinner. Or, someone may need two to three snacks each day. Look at your food diary to determine your general food guidelines, or have your dietitian help you determine them and give you more options for each meal.

Plate Methods

The plate method is a visual method for teaching food amounts. If you are feeling overwhelmed, or just need something fairly easy to monitor your portion sizes, this method can help you. Take out one of your dinner plates and divide it in half. You fill one half with vegetables. The other half is divided into two sections—one for starchy foods and the other for protein foods.

There are several variations of this method, all dividing a plate and using the sections to guide food amounts. It is a quick method to learn and encourages eating a variety of food in limited amounts.

The First Step in Diabetes Meal Planning

This meal planning method has you select the number of servings you would like to eat each day from the six food groups listed in the following Food Groups table. Then you divide those servings throughout the day into your meals and snacks. An example of the First-Step Food Plan shows one meal plan based on this method (see page 47).

First Step in Diabetes Meal Planning Guidelines

- Eat meals and snacks at regular times every day.
- Eat about the same amount of food each day.
- Try not to skip meals.
- If you want to lose weight, cut down on your portion size. If you skip a meal, you may eat too much at your next meal.
- Eat a wide variety of foods every day. Try new foods.
- Eat high-fiber foods, such as fruits, vegetables, grains, and beans.
- Use less added fat, sugar, and salt.

Your blood glucose checks will guide you in making changes in how your food is distributed throughout a day.

Food Groups Using the Diabetes Food Guide Pyramid*

Food Group	Examples of Food and Serving Size Appropriate for a Person Who Has Diabetes	Notes
Grains, beans, and starchy vegetables (6 or more servings per day)	1 slice of bread ½ small bagel, English muffin, or pita bread (1 oz) ½ small hamburger or hot dog bun (1 oz) 1 tortilla, 6-inch 4 to 6 crackers ½ cup cooked cereal or bulgur ⅓ cup cooked rice or pasta ¾ cup dry cereal ½ cup cooked beans, lentils, peas, or corn 1 small potato 1 cup winter squash ½ cup sweet potato or yam	• Choose whole-grain foods such as whole-grain bread or crackers, tortillas, bran cereal, brown rice, or bulgur. They're nutritious and high in fiber. • Choose beans as a good source of fiber. • Use whole-wheat or other whole-grain flours in cooking and baking. • Eat more low-fat breads such as bagels, tortillas, English muffins, and pita bread. • For snacks, try pretzels or low-fat crackers.
Fruits (2–4 servings per day)	1 small fresh fruit ½ cup canned fruit ¼ cup dried fruit ½ cup fruit juice	• Choose whole fruits more often than juices. They have more fiber. • Choose fruits and fruit juices without added sweeteners or syrups. • Choose citrus fruit such as oranges, grapefruit, or tangerines every day.
Nonstarchy vegetables (3–5 servings per day)	1 cup raw vegetables ½ cup cooked vegetables ½ cup tomato or vegetable juice	• Choose fresh or frozen vegetables without added sauces, fats, or salt. • Choose more dark green and deep yellow vegetables, such as spinach, broccoli, romaine, carrots, chilies, and peppers.

(continued)

Food Groups Using the Diabetes Food Guide Pyramid *(continued)*

Food Group	Examples of Food and Serving Size	Notes
Milk (2–3 servings per day)	1 cup milk $^2/_3$ cup yogurt	• Choose low-fat or nonfat milk or yogurt. Yogurt has natural sugar in it. It can also have added sugar or artificial sweeteners. Yogurt with artificial sweeteners has fewer calories than yogurt with added sugar.
Meat and Substitutes (2–3 servings per day)	2–3 oz cooked lean meat, poultry, or fish ½ cup tuna or ¾ cup cottage cheese† 2–3 oz cheese 1 egg† 2 tablespoons peanut butter† 4 oz tofu†	• Choose fish and poultry more often. Remove the skin from chicken and turkey. • Select lean cuts of beef, veal, pork, or wild game. • Trim all visible fat from meat. Bake, roast, broil, grill, or boil instead of frying or adding fat. • Select reduced-fat cheese.
Fats and sweets	Fats: 2 tablespoons avocado 1 tablespoon cream cheese or salad dressing 1 teaspoon butter, margarine, oil, or mayonnaise 10 peanuts	• Eat less fat. • Eat less saturated fat. It is found in meat and animal products such as hamburger, cheese, bacon, and butter. Saturated fat is usually solid at room temperature.
	Sweets: ½ cup ice cream 1 small cupcake or muffin 2 small cookies	• Choose sweets less often because they're high in fat and sugar. When you do eat sweets, make them part of your healthy diet. Substitute them for other foods in your food plan with equal amounts of carbohydrate. Don't eat them as extras.

*Based on the diabetes food guide pyramid adapted from the USDA Food Guide Pyramid. Servings sizes are similar to the servings in the diabetes exchange list and provide about 15 grams of carbohydrate.

†Same as 1 oz meat.

Source: The First Step in Diabetes Meal Planning, American Diabetes Association and American Dietetic Association, Chicago, Illinois, 2003; used with permission.

Example of a First-Step Food Plan

	Total servings each day	Meal or snack time			
		8:00 A.M.	12:00 P.M.	6:00 P.M.	9:00 P.M.
Grains, beans, and starchy vegetables	10	2	3	3	2
Vegetables	4–5		2	2–3	
Fruits	3		1	1	1
Milk	2	1		1	
Meat and others	2–3	0–1	1 (2–3 oz)	1 (2–3 oz)	
Fats and sweets	3–4	0–1	1	2	

Calorie Counting Plans

Another way to establish a pattern of food intake is to count calories if you are on a weight loss or weight maintenance plan. You may have a set amount of calories that you eat for each meal or a total for a day. For example, you may want to limit your calories to 1,500 a day so you could plan on having 500 calories at each meal. Often establishing a range of calories gives you a little more flexibility but enough structure to achieve your weight goals.

A calorie counting plan could look like this:

- Breakfast: 300–400 calories
- Lunch: 400–500 calories
- Dinner: 400–500 calories
- Snack: Calories left to total 1,500 for the day

This type of plan may be very successful for you. Check your blood glucose levels to determine if you need to also monitor your carbohydrate intake. The carbohydrate counting plan below describes how you can do that. You may want to alternate between the two plans so you can benefit from the advantages of each.

Carbohydrate Counting Plans

Foods that affect the blood glucose level the most are those high in carbohydrate (starches and sugars) and include breads, cereals, pasta, grains, milk, and fruit. This is the newest diabetes meal planning method and focuses mainly on carbohydrates, by counting the amount of carbohydrates consumed at each meal and snack. It is very useful once you begin to take a diabetes medication and is most useful if you use flexible insulin management (three to four injections a day) or an insulin pump. It is explained in more detail in chapter 14.

Exchange System Plans

In the exchange system, food is categorized into six food groups similar to those found in the food guide pyramid as outlined in the table on pages 45–46. Each food in a particular group is given a serving size, so each serving has a similar amount of carbohydrate, protein, and fat. For example, on average, a single serving of vegetables provides 5 grams of carbohydrate, 2 grams of protein, no fat, and 25 calories. Because each serving is similar, you can exchange or trade one serving of one food for a serving of another food within the same food group. See chapter 15 for more details.

STICKING TO YOUR FOOD PLAN—AND MAKING SURE IT MEETS YOUR NEEDS

Begin with a food plan that is easy to follow. A registered dietitian is the person to best help you with this. She can help at any step in the process—reviewing your eating patterns, helping you know what your usual carbohydrate intake amounts are, discussing what changes might be easiest for you to make to reach your goals, and helping you make decisions about changes based on what you want to do. She will also help you review your food plan with your blood glucose monitoring records so you can evaluate the timing of your meals and how much you eat. This is the next step in designing your food plan—being sure it is the best for you and your diabetes.

CHAPTER 5

Making Quick and Easy Meals

T his chapter will:

- Provide tips for preparing quick meals
- Give you menu ideas
- Discuss how to get the most food for your allotted calories
- Describe how holiday and special occasion meals fit a diabetes food plan

PLANNING AHEAD AND CREATING A VARIETY OF MEALS

There are two steps to help make meal planning a snap. First, take time each week to plan your meals so you know in advance what you will be eating. Second, have the ingredients you need for making the meals. Meal planning should not be that difficult. What makes it difficult is that most people don't plan ahead. In fact, many people don't know what they are having for dinner until it is almost time to eat.

Start planning your meals by thinking about your favorite meals. Write down three to five of your favorite breakfasts, lunches, and dinners, then fill in the rest of the week with other meals, or repeat some of your favorites. This will take 15–30 minutes. Your food plan will guide you in knowing how much of each food to eat. If you are not sure, the guidelines in chapter 4 will help you, or ask your dietitian for assistance. Post your list of menus on your refrigerator or another handy place so you are quickly reminded about your menus. This list of menus will help you plan your shopping list.

It's important to have on hand some staple ingredients to make a quick meal when you don't want your preplanned meal, you are feeling rushed, or you have little energy to prepare a meal. A well-stocked kitchen and a list of quick meal options allow you to easily follow your food plan when time is tight. Preplanning meals is the key and provides great opportunities for a variety of quick meals.

SIX QUICK MEAL IDEAS

Following are six quick meal suggestions that can be eaten any time—breakfast, lunch, or dinner. Adjust the portion sizes for your calorie and carbohydrate needs, and choose a beverage that fits your food plan such as milk, water, or iced tea. You can copy this list and tape it to a kitchen cabinet for quick reference; be sure to add some of your own suggestions.

- Hot or cold cereal with milk and a piece of fresh fruit
- French toast topped with reduced-sugar applesauce or grated cheese, and sliced fruit
- Peanut butter sandwich and vegetable sticks such as celery, broccoli, and peppers
- Low-fat frozen meal and carrot sticks
- Pasta with chicken or tofu, tossed with cooked vegetables
- Tortilla filled with canned beans, salsa, lettuce, and tomato

INGREDIENTS FOR QUICK MEALS

It is easy to make a quick meal when you have the ingredients readily available. If your refrigerator and cupboards are almost empty or contain the wrong foods, you are facing a challenge. Keep a well-stocked kitchen. Fill your kitchen cupboards with a supply of lower calorie staples like the following to make it easy to fix a quick meal that fits your food plan:

Grains, beans, and starchy vegetables
- Sandwich breads, bagels, pita bread, or English muffins
- Soft corn tortillas or low-fat flour tortillas
- Low-fat, low-sodium crackers
- Plain cereal, hot or cold
- Plain pasta
- Brown and white (quick) rice
- Canned beans and peas
- Low-fat popcorn
- Pretzels

Fruits
- Fresh, frozen, or canned fruits in light syrup or juice

Vegetables
- Plain fresh, frozen, or no-salt-added canned vegetables
- Low-sodium tomato sauce or tomato paste

Dairy foods
- Fat-free or low-fat milk, yogurt, cheeses, and cottage cheese

Meat, poultry, fish, and other protein
- Whole eggs or egg substitute
- Frozen boneless, skinless white meat of chicken or turkey
- Frozen lean ground turkey
- Frozen or canned fish and shellfish

- Frozen beef: round, sirloin, chuck arm, loin, and extra-lean ground beef
- Frozen pork: leg, shoulder, or tenderloin
- Frozen veal: shoulder, ground veal, cutlets, or sirloin
- Peanut butter
- Tofu

Fats

- Light or diet margarine, tub or liquid
- Low-fat or nonfat salad dressings and mayonnaise
- Vegetable oils

Sweets

- Jam and jelly (reduced sugar)
- Low-fat cookies, such as animal crackers, graham crackers, vanilla wafers, fig bars, or ginger snaps
- Angel food cake

Other

- Mustard and low-sodium ketchup
- Herbs and spices
- Salsa
- Low-sodium soy sauce

SHOPPING FOR YOUR MEALS

You can use the previous list to take stock of your kitchen. Check-mark those items you are missing and then take the list with you when shopping so you buy what you need. Also add the ingredients you will need to prepare the meals you have planned for the week. Without a list, the whole shopping experience can be overwhelming and frustrating—a maze of confusing shelves of foods. Three guiding principles of grocery shopping are: (1) always have a shopping list and buy only what is on your list, (2) avoid crowds to make the trip less hectic, and (3) do not shop when you are hungry.

Most grocery stores are laid out similarly, with foods grouped together in sections by food categories and method of processing—fresh, canned, or frozen. The sections correspond to the six food groups in the Food Guide Pyramid (grains, beans, and starchy vegetables; fruits; nonstarchy vegetables; milk; meat and meat subtitutes; and fats and sweets; see pages 45 and 46) and can be used to organize your shopping list. You can organize your shopping list by the six food group categories, then write fresh, canned, and frozen in each of the categories. This can help you be more efficient when shopping and save you from making extra trips to the grocery store to get what you may have forgotten.

Dietetic Foods

Often there is one area of a grocery store containing foods reduced in calories, sugar, and/or sodium. People with diabetes often gravitate to this area thinking those are the food items they must eat. Some of these foods may be helpful in your diabetes food plan, but they are often not necessary. Other similar items may be found throughout the store, and may be less expensive. For example, brands of reduced-sugar canned fruits are stocked with other canned fruits, low-calorie sweeteners are usually located near the white and brown sugars, and low-sodium foods are often displayed with other similar foods containing more sodium.

Reading the nutrition facts panel on the food label (see chapter 16) will help guide you in making the decision as to whether a particular food is appropriate for you, and how it fits into your food plan. If you choose reduced-calorie or sugar-free foods, be sure to check their carbohydrate content, as they may be "dietetic" and "suitable for diabetes" but are often not "free" foods. Usually most foods can be part of a food plan, but must be counted and balanced with your other food choices.

Liquid Meals and Bars

A number of manufacturers have responded to people's busy, hectic lifestyles by producing and selling liquid meals and bars that replace meals. These foods are often highly fortified with vitamins and minerals, and sometimes with antioxidants and fiber.

Are these meal replacements valuable in a diabetes food plan? Meal replacements are as valuable to the person with diabetes as those without diabetes. In a crunch, they can provide needed nutrition. Certainly, they don't replace the value of a well-rounded meal high in whole grains, fruits, and vegetables. Yet there are times when a very quick simple meal is needed and these meal replacements can provide that.

Let the nutrition information on the package guide you. Look at the values most important to your food plan such as total carbohydrate, calories, fat, and sodium. Also look for meal replacements that contain fiber. You may need to supplement the meal replacement with a piece of fruit or glass of milk to meet your carbohydrate needs.

MENUS FOR SPECIAL OCCASIONS

Throughout the year you will participate in a number of special occasions, such as birthdays and Thanksgiving, that call for special foods. By thinking through these situations and knowing, or anticipating, what foods will be available, you will be able to make decisions that will accommodate your diabetes and allow you to enjoy these special events.

Finding out the time frame for the special occasion will help you decide whether you need to adjust your mealtime. If you can, also find out what food is going to be served so you will be able to determine how it will fit into your food plan. For example, you may be invited to a birthday party that includes a dinner that will be served at your usual mealtime, and cake and ice cream served later in the evening. This is the information you need to know to make an adjustment in your food intake.

There are a number of options for such an occasion, including eating less at dinner in order to have a small serving of cake and ice cream; skipping the cake and ice cream but requesting a calorie-free beverage; having the regular dinner and the cake and ice cream and going for a walk between the two or after the cake. If you take rapid-acting insulin, you could take an extra small amount of insulin based on your insulin to carbohydrate ratio (discussed in chapter 14) before you eat the cake and ice cream to cover the extra carbohydrate. The option that is best for you will depend on the type of diabetes you have, how it is treated, and what your diabetes goals are. Discuss these types of situations with your diabetes care team before they happen so you can be prepared.

Also, for many special occasions, you may feel comfortable bringing an appetizer or a dish to share. Consider bringing something that you know will fit easily into your meal plan. This may be a vegetable platter with low-calorie dressing, a hot vegetable dish like steamed broccoli or asparagus, low-fat cheesecake, or fresh fruit with low-calorie frozen whipped topping.

ADJUSTING RECIPES

You may want to include family recipes in your diabetes food plan for everyday meals or special occasions. Sometimes these recipes will need a little tweaking to help them better fit your food plan. Common changes include reducing the amount of fat, sugar, or sodium in the recipe.

Reducing Fat and Sugar

To reduce the fat in a food you may need to adjust how you cook a food, or just use less fat while cooking. Some suggestions are as follows:

- Cut back on fat by using a different cooking method: bake, broil, steam, poach, or grill foods instead of frying or cooking in fat. Broiling and grilling allow fat to drip away from the food.
- Reduce fat by using less when sautéing, or when making a sauce or dressing.
- When making stews or soups ahead of time, refrigerate them and then skim off the hard fat on top.
- Replace fat used to coat baking pans with a nonstick cooking spray or parchment paper when possible.
- Use nonfat spreads like spicy mustard and horseradish on sandwiches, and replace cheese with lettuce, tomato, sprouts, or cucumbers.

Appendix F lists some common ingredient substitutions to lower the fat and sugar content in foods.

Boosting Flavors

When reducing the fat, sugar, or sodium in a recipe, you may need to boost the flavor in other ways to compensate for the taste changes. Consider the following, especially when reducing the sodium in a food (adapted from Powers, MA; Hendley, J: *Forbidden Foods Diabetic Cooking*, American Diabetes Association, Alexandria, Virginia, 2000):

- Use fresh herbs, specialty spices, and pure flavoring extracts when available, because their flavors are more intense.
- Increase the amount of other spices already in the recipe.
- Add seasonings at the right time during the cooking process. Often basil and other fresh herbs are more flavorful when added towards the end of the cooking time. Add dried, delicate herbs like chervil or marjoram later in the cooking process. Some examples of spices that should be added earlier, so their flavors will develop more, are cumin, coriander, allspice, nutmeg, and ginger.

• Select seasonings that will enhance flavors that are already in the recipe. For example nutmeg goes well with the buttery flavor of creamy dishes, and fresh chopped parsley, which is delicious in tomato-based dishes and soups, brings out the flavors of other dried herbs.

The goal of any recipe is to have the food taste great. For this reason, you will probably not be able to omit all the fat, sugar, and sodium, yet you will be able to make some adjustments to make it fit your food plan better. Even with adjustments, "diabetes" recipes should still be so tasty that you, your family, and your guests will enjoy them.

CHOOSING SNACKS

Most people with diabetes do not need snacks. If you do eat snacks, you may need to have less food at meals so that your calories balance out throughout the day. If you prefer smaller meals, you may need snacks. Choose snacks that complement your meals and provide healthy nutrients. For example, if you don't like fruit with meals, then fruit may make a great snack option for you.

To decide if you need to have a snack, review your blood glucose records. Is there a time of the day when your blood glucose level is consistently lower than you would like? A snack may help prevent this. Since low-blood-glucose episodes are often related to certain diabetes medications, adjusting the medication may also prevent the low-blood-glucose episode without requiring a snack to be added. Discuss this with your health team.

If you need to have a snack, you may wonder about the specialty snack bars that claim to be "slow-release glucose" or to "reduce the risk of hypoglycemia." They may, in fact, cause a slower and lower rise in blood glucose, so don't use them to treat a low-blood-glucose reaction.

You can "test" their effect to see if they offer you any advantages in reducing a post-meal blood glucose rise or preventing low blood glucose. Do this test particularly if you eat a nighttime snack to prevent low blood glucose during the night. Check your blood glucose before you consume the bar, then two, three, and four hours after. Compare these results with those of other foods you might have for a bedtime snack. You may find that a simple snack of fruit, crackers, popcorn, or leftovers is just as effective in maintaining your target blood glucose goals.

A WEEK OF MENU IDEAS

If you need ideas for breakfast, lunch, or dinner—for a whole day, or for a week—the following menus will help. (If the print size of the menus is too small to read comfortably, you may enlarge the section that has your calorie level at a photocopier.) To use these menus, you need to know how many calories you need each day. If you are not sure, use the guidelines in chapter 8 to figure out your basic calorie needs. If you are counting carbohydrates, they are listed in parentheses after certain foods in the menus.

A variety of menu options are included—some with meat, some without, and covering various ethnic choices. Choose the menus that fit your food preferences and feel free to mix and match menus from the seven days.

Each menu provides about 50% of calories from carbohydrate, 20% from protein, and 30% from fat. The food is distributed throughout the day according to the distribution described on page 67. Both the calorie and food distributions are fairly common, but may not correspond with your eating style or food plan, so feel free to move food to the meal or snack time that fits your needs. (Ideally, design your own personal food plan with a dietitian, then adjust the food amounts to fit your plan.) See chapters 10 and 14 for more information on carbohydrate distribution.

Sample Menu Plan—Day 1

1,200 kcal (9 carbs)

Breakfast:
½ cup oatmeal (1)
1 small banana (1)
8 fl oz skim milk (1)

Lunch:
2 slices light bread (1)
2 oz low-fat cheese
3 tsp margarine
1 cup tomato soup (1)
½ cup peaches (1)
Mineral water

Dinner:
1 6-inch flour tortilla (1)
½ cup black beans (1)
½ cup peppers/onions
¼ cup salsa
2 oz low-fat cheese
½ cup fruit cocktail (1)
8 fl oz skim milk (1)

1,500 kcal (12 carbs)

Breakfast:
½ cup oatmeal (1)
1 small banana (1)
8 fl oz skim milk (1)
1 small muffin (1)
1 tsp margarine

Lunch:
2 slices light bread (1)
2 oz low-fat cheese
3 tsp margarine
2 cups tomato soup (2)
½ cup peaches (1)
Mineral water

Dinner:
1 6-inch flour tortilla (1)
½ cup black beans (1)
½ cup peppers/onions
¼ cup salsa
2 oz low-fat cheese
½ cup fruit cocktail (1)
8 fl oz skim milk (1)

1,800 kcal (14 carbs)

Breakfast:
½ cup oatmeal (1)
1 small banana (1)
8 fl oz skim milk (1)
1 small muffin (1)
1 tsp margarine

Lunch:
2 slices light bread (1)
2 oz low-fat cheese
3 tsp margarine
2 cups tomato soup (2)
1 cup peaches (2)
Mineral water

Dinner:
2 6-inch flour tortilla (2)
2 oz chicken
½ cup black beans (1)
1 cup peppers/onions
¼ cup salsa
2 oz low-fat cheese
½ cup fruit cocktail (1)
8 fl oz skim milk (1)

2,000 kcal (16 carbs)

Breakfast:
½ cup oatmeal (1)
1 small banana (1)
8 fl oz skim milk (1)
1 small muffin (1)
1 tsp margarine

Lunch:
2 slices bread (2)
2 oz low-fat cheese
3 tsp margarine
1 cup tomato soup (1)
1 cup peaches (2)
Mineral water

Dinner:
2 6-inch flour tortilla (2)
2 oz chicken
½ cup black beans (1)
1 cup peppers/onions
¼ cup salsa
2 oz low-fat cheese
½ cup fruit cocktail (1)
8 fl oz skim milk (1)

Snack:
8 fl oz skim milk (1)
5 vanilla wafers (1)

2,500 kcal (20 carbs)

Breakfast:
½ cup oatmeal (1)
1 small banana (1)
8 fl oz skim milk (1)
1 small muffin (1)
1 tsp margarine

Lunch:
2 slices bread (2)
2 oz low-fat cheese
3 tsp margarine
2 oz ham
1 cup tomato soup (1)
6 saltine crackers (1)
1 cup peaches (2)
½ cup broccoli
½ cup cauliflower
2 Tbsp ranch dip
Mineral water

Dinner:
2 6-inch flour tortilla (2)
2 oz chicken
½ cup black beans (1)
⅓ cup rice (1)
1 cup peppers/onions
¼ cup salsa
2 oz low-fat cheese
½ cup fruit cocktail (1)
8 fl oz skim milk (1)

Snacks:
8 fl oz skim milk (1)
5 vanilla wafers (1)

1 oz tortilla chips (1)
½ cup pineapple bits (1)
¼ cup salsa

Sample Menu Plan—Day 2

1,200 kcal (9 carbs)

Breakfast:
1 slice wheat toast (1)
2 tsp sugar-free jelly
1 tsp margarine
1 cup low-fat yogurt (1)
½ cup orange juice (1)
Coffee or tea

Lunch:
1 cup mix salad greens
3 oz grilled chicken
1 oz low-fat cheese
1 Tbsp dressing
½ cup croutons (1)
1 dinner roll (1)
1 tsp margarine
1 peach (1)
8 fl oz skim milk (1)

Dinner:
⅔ cup pasta noodles (2)
¼ cup zucchini
¼ cup eggplant
½ cup pasta sauce (1)
½ cup unsweetened
  applesauce (1)
Mineral water

1,500 kcal (12 carbs)

Breakfast:
2 slices wheat toast (2)
4 tsp sugar-free jelly
2 tsp margarine
1 cup low-fat yogurt (1)
½ cup orange juice (1)
Coffee or tea

Lunch:
2 cups mix salad greens
4 oz grilled chicken
2 oz low-fat cheese
1 Tbsp dressing
½ cup croutons (1)
2 dinner rolls (2)
1 tsp margarine
1 peach (1)
8 fl oz skim milk (1)

Dinner:
⅔ cup pasta noodles (2)
¼ cup zucchini
¼ cup eggplant
1 breadstick (1)
½ cup pasta sauce (1)
½ cup unsweetened
  applesauce (1)
Mineral water

1,800 kcal (14 carbs)

Breakfast:
2 slices wheat toast (2)
4 tsp sugar-free jelly
2 tsp margarine
1 cup low-fat yogurt (1)
½ cup orange juice (1)
Coffee or tea

Lunch:
2 cups mix salad greens
4 oz grilled chicken
2 oz low-fat cheese
1 Tbsp dressing
½ cup croutons (1)
2 dinner rolls (2)
1 tsp margarine
1 peach (1)
8 fl oz skim milk (1)

Dinner:
⅔ cup pasta noodles (2)
¼ cup zucchini
¼ cup eggplant
½ cup pasta sauce (1)
1 breadstick (1)
½ cup unsweetened
  applesauce (1)
Mineral water

Snack:
8 fl oz skim milk (1)
1 piece coffeecake (1)

2,500 kcal (20 carbs)

Breakfast:
2 slices wheat toast (2)
4 tsp sugar-free jelly
2 tsp margarine
1 cup low-fat yogurt (1)
½ cup orange juice (1)
Coffee or tea

Lunch:
2 cups mix salad greens
4 oz grilled chicken
2 oz low-fat cheese
¾ cup diced tomatoes
¼ cup diced onions
1 Tbsp dressing
½ cup croutons (1)
2 dinner rolls (2)
1 tsp margarine
2 peach (1)
8 fl oz skim milk (1)

Dinner:
⅔ cup pasta noodles (2)
½ cup zucchini
½ cup eggplant
2 oz sirloin strips
½ cup pasta sauce (2)
1 breadstick (1)
½ cup unsweetened
  applesauce (1)
Mineral water

Snacks:
8 fl oz skim milk (1)
1 piece coffeecake (1)

½ cup frozen yogurt (1)
1¼ cups strawberries (1)

61

Sample Menu Plan—Day 3

1,200 kcal (9 carbs)

Breakfast:
½ cup TOTAL cereal (1)
8 fl oz skim milk (1)
½ cup apple juice (1)

Lunch:
2 slices wheat bread (2)
2 oz turkey
4 tsp mayo
2 lettuce leaves
3 tomato slices
1 apple (1)
Diet soda

Dinner:
3 oz sirloin steak
Small baked potato (1)
1 tsp margarine
2 Tbsp sour cream
1 cup green beans
1 dinner roll (1)
1 tsp margarine
½ cup unsweetened
  applesauce (1)
8 fl oz skim milk (1)

1,500 kcal (12 carbs)

Breakfast:
1 cup TOTAL cereal (2)
8 fl oz skim milk (1)
½ cup apple juice (1)

Lunch:
2 slices wheat bread (2)
2 oz turkey
4 tsp mayo
2 lettuce leaves
3 tomato slices
1 apple (1)
3 gingersnaps (1)
1 cup carrot sticks
2 Tbsp dip
Diet soda

Dinner:
3 oz sirloin steak
Small baked potato (1)
1 tsp margarine
2 Tbsp sour cream
1 cup green beans
1 dinner roll (1)
1 tsp margarine
½ cup unsweetened
  applesauce (1)
8 fl oz skim milk (1)

1,800 kcal (14 carbs)

Breakfast:
1 cup TOTAL cereal (2)
8 fl oz skim milk (1)
½ cup apple juice (1)

Lunch:
2 slices wheat bread (2)
3 oz turkey
4 tsp mayo
2 lettuce leaves
3 tomato slices
1 apple (1)
6 gingersnaps (2)
1 cup carrot sticks
2 Tbsp dip
10 peanuts
Diet soda

Dinner:
3 oz sirloin steak
Small baked potato (1)
1 tsp margarine
2 Tbsp sour cream
1 cup green beans
2 dinner rolls (2)
2 tsp margarine
½ cup unsweetened
  applesauce (1)
8 fl oz skim milk (1)

2,000 kcal (16 carbs)

Breakfast:
1 cup TOTAL cereal (2)
8 fl oz skim milk (1)
½ cup apple juice (1)

Lunch:
2 slices wheat bread (2)
3 oz turkey
4 tsp mayo
2 lettuce leaves
3 tomato slices
1 apple (1)
6 gingersnaps (2)
1 cup carrot sticks
2 Tbsp dip
10 peanuts
Diet soda

Dinner:
3 oz sirloin steak
Small baked potato (1)
1 tsp margarine
2 Tbsp sour cream
1 cup green beans
2 dinner rolls (2)
2 tsp margarine
½ cup unsweetened
  applesauce (1)
8 fl oz skim milk (1)

Snack:
1 cup low-fat yogurt (1)
¾ cup blueberries (1)

2,500 kcal (20 carbs)

Breakfast:
1 cup TOTAL cereal (2)
8 fl oz skim milk (1)
½ cup apple juice (1)

Lunch:
2 slices wheat bread (2)
3 oz turkey
2 oz low-fat cheese
4 tsp mayo
2 lettuce leaves
3 tomato slices
1 apple (1)
1 orange (1)
6 gingersnaps (2)
1 cup carrot sticks
2 Tbsp dip
10 peanuts
Diet soda

Dinner:
3 oz sirloin steak
½ cup mushrooms/onions
Large baked potato (2)
1 tsp margarine
4 Tbsp sour cream
1 cup green beans
2 dinner rolls (2)
2 tsp margarine
½ cup unsweetened
  applesauce (1)
8 fl oz skim milk (1)

Snacks:
1 cup low-fat yogurt (1)
¾ cup blueberries (1)

2 Tbsp raisins (1)
¾ oz trail mix (1)

62

Sample Menu Plan—Day 4

1,200 kcal (9 carbs)

Breakfast:
1 4½-inch waffle (1)
2 Tbsp light syrup
1 tsp margarine
1 cup yogurt (1)
¾ cup blackberries (1)
Coffee or tea

Lunch:
½ cup chili w/beans (1)
6 saltine crackers (1)
½ cup broccoli
½ cup cauliflower
1 Tbsp dip
1 apple (1)
Diet soda

Dinner:
4 oz hamburger
1 hamburger bun (2)
2 lettuce leaves
2 tomato slices
1 Tbsp ketchup
1¼ cup watermelon (1)
3 fl oz skim milk (1)

1,500 kcal (12 carbs)

Breakfast:
2 4½-inch waffles (2)
4 Tbsp light syrup
2 tsp margarine
1 cup yogurt (1)
¾ cup blackberries (1)
Coffee or tea

Lunch:
1 cup chili w/beans (2)
12 saltine crackers (2)
½ cup broccoli
½ cup cauliflower
2 Tbsp dip
1 apple (1)
Diet soda

Dinner:
4 oz hamburger
1 hamburger bun (2)
2 lettuce leaves
2 tomato slices
1 Tbsp ketchup
1¼ cup watermelon (1)
1 oz chips (1)
1 cup celery sticks
2 tsp peanut butter
8 fl oz skim milk (1)

1,800 kcal (14 carbs)

Breakfast:
2 4½-inch waffles (2)
4 Tbsp light syrup
2 tsp margarine
1 cup yogurt (1)
¾ cup blackberries (1)
Coffee or tea

Lunch:
1 cup chili w/beans (2)
12 saltine crackers (2)
½ cup broccoli
½ cup cauliflower
2 Tbsp dip
1 apple (1)
Diet soda

Dinner:
4 oz hamburger
1 hamburger bun (2)
2 lettuce leaves
2 tomato slices
1 Tbsp ketchup
1¼ cup watermelon (1)
1 oz chips (1)
1 cup celery sticks
2 tsp peanut butter
8 fl oz skim milk (1)

Snack:
1 cup sugar-free pudding (2)

2,000 kcal (16 carbs)

Breakfast:
2 4½-inch waffles (2)
4 Tbsp light syrup
2 tsp margarine
1 cup yogurt (1)
¾ cup blackberries (1)
Coffee or tea

Lunch:
1 cup chili w/beans (2)
12 saltine crackers (2)
½ cup broccoli
½ cup cauliflower
2 Tbsp dip
1 apple (1)
Diet soda

Dinner:
4 oz hamburger
1 hamburger bun (2)
2 lettuce leaves
2 tomato slices
1 Tbsp ketchup
1¼ cup watermelon (1)
1 oz chips (1)
1 cup celery sticks
2 tsp peanut butter
8 fl oz skim milk (1)

Snack:
1 cup sugar-free pudding (2)

2,500 kcal (20 carbs)

Breakfast:
2 4½-inch waffles (2)
4 Tbsp light syrup
2 tsp margarine
1 cup yogurt (1)
¾ cup blackberries (1)
Coffee or tea

Lunch:
1 cup chili w/beans (2)
12 saltine crackers (2)
½ cup broccoli
½ cup cauliflower
2 Tbsp dip
1 apple (1)
1 banana (1)
Diet soda

Dinner:
4 oz hamburger
1 hamburger bun (2)
2 lettuce leaves
2 tomato slices
1 Tbsp ketchup
1¼ cup watermelon (1)
1 oz chips (2)
1 cup celery sticks
2 tsp peanut butter
8 fl oz skim milk (1)

Snacks:
1 cup sugar-free pudding (2)
2 oz string cheese
¾ oz pretzels (1)
½ cup fruit juice (1)

Sample Menu Plan—Day 5

1,200 kcal (9 carbs)
Breakfast:
1 scrambled egg
1 buttermilk biscuit (1)
1 tsp margarine
½ grapefruit, sections (1)
8 fl oz skim milk (1)

Lunch:
1 cup macaroni & cheese (2)
½ cup carrot sticks
½ cup celery sticks
2 Tbsp dip
1 cup melon (1)
Diet soda

Dinner:
½ cup red beans and rice (1)
2 oz cornbread (1)
½ cup cooked greens
1 tsp olive oil
½ cup canned peaches (1)
8 fl oz skim milk (1)

1,500 kcal (12 carbs)
Breakfast:
1 scrambled egg
1 buttermilk biscuit (1)
1 tsp margarine
½ grapefruit, sections (1)
8 fl oz skim milk (1)

Lunch:
1 cup macaroni & cheese (2)
1 dinner roll (1)
1 tsp margarine
½ cup carrot sticks
½ cup celery sticks
2 Tbsp dip
1 cup melon (1)
Diet soda

Dinner:
½ cup red beans and rice (1)
2 oz cornbread (1)
1 tsp margarine
½ cup cooked greens
1 tsp olive oil
½ cup canned peaches (1)
8 fl oz skim milk (1)

1,800 kcal (14 carbs)
Breakfast:
1 scrambled egg
1 buttermilk biscuit (1)
1 tsp margarine
1 turkey sausage link
½ grapefruit, sections (1)
1 small orange, sections (1)
8 fl oz skim milk (1)

Lunch:
1½ cups macaroni & cheese (3)
1 dinner roll (1)
1 tsp margarine
½ cup carrot sticks
½ cup celery sticks
2 Tbsp dip
1 cup melon (1)
Diet soda

Dinner:
½ cup red beans and rice (1)
2 oz cornbread (1)
1 tsp margarine
½ cup cooked greens
1 tsp olive oil
½ cup canned peaches (1)
8 fl oz skim milk (1)

2,000 kcal (16 carbs)
Breakfast:
1 scrambled egg
1 buttermilk biscuit (1)
1 tsp margarine
1 turkey sausage link
½ grapefruit, sections (1)
1 small orange, sections (1)
8 fl oz skim milk (1)

Lunch:
1½ cups macaroni & cheese (3)
1 dinner roll (1)
1 tsp margarine
½ cup carrot sticks
½ cup celery sticks
2 Tbsp dip
1 cup melon (1)
Diet soda

Dinner:
1 cup red beans and rice (2)
2 oz cornbread (1)
1 tsp margarine
1½ cup cooked greens
1 tsp olive oil
½ cup canned peaches (1)
8 fl oz skim milk (1)

Snack:
½ cup regular pudding (2)

2,500 kcal (20 carbs)
Breakfast:
2 scrambled eggs
1 buttermilk biscuit (1)
1 tsp margarine
1 turkey sausage link
½ grapefruit, sections (1)
1 small orange, sections (1)
8 fl oz skim milk (1)

Lunch:
1½ cups macaroni & cheese (3)
1 dinner roll (1)
1 tsp margarine
½ cup carrot sticks
½ cup celery sticks
2 Tbsp dip
2 cup melon (2)
Diet soda

Dinner:
1½ cup red beans and rice (3)
2 oz cornbread (1)
1 tsp margarine
1½ cup cooked greens
1 tsp olive oil
½ cup canned peaches (1)
8 fl oz skim milk (1)

Snacks:
½ cup regular pudding (2)

1 oatmeal raisin cookie (1)
8 fl oz skim milk (1)

Sample Menu Plan—Day 6

1,200 kcal (9 carbs)
Breakfast:
1 cup low-fat yogurt (1)
¾ cup boysenberries (1)
¼ cup granola (1)
Coffee or tea

Lunch:
¼ cup cottage cheese
½ cup mango slices (1)
½ cup pear slices (1)
1 dinner roll (1)
1 tsp margarine
Tea or water

Dinner:
3 oz roasted pork
1 cup rice (3)
1 cup veggie stir-fry
1 tsp stir-fry sauce
1 tsp peanut oil
1 cup low-fat yogurt (1)
Tea or water

1,500 kcal (12 carbs)
Breakfast:
1 cup low-fat yogurt (1)
¾ cup boysenberries (1)
¼ cup granola (1)
½ cup pineapple juice (1)
Coffee or tea

Lunch:
¼ cup cottage cheese
½ cup mango slices (1)
½ cup pear slices (1)
2 dinner rolls (2)
2 tsp margarine
Tea or water

Dinner:
3 oz roasted pork
1 cup rice (3)
1 cup veggie stir-fry
2 tsp stir-fry sauce
2 tsp peanut oil
1 cup low-fat yogurt (1)
Tea or water

1,800 kcal (14 carbs)
Breakfast:
1 cup low-fat yogurt (1)
¾ cup boysenberries (1)
¼ cup granola (1)
½ cup pineapple juice (1)
Coffee or tea

Lunch:
1 cup cottage cheese
½ cup mango slices (1)
½ cup pear slices (1)
2 dinner rolls (2)
2 tsp margarine
3 graham crackers (1)
Tea or water

Dinner:
3 oz roasted pork
1 cup rice (3)
1 cup veggie stir-fry
2 tsp stir-fry sauce
2 tsp peanut oil
1 cup low-fat yogurt (1)
2 fortune cookies (1)
Tea or water

2,000 kcal (16 carbs)
Breakfast:
1 cup low-fat yogurt (1)
¾ cup boysenberries (1)
¼ cup granola (1)
½ cup pineapple juice (1)
Coffee or tea

Lunch:
1 cup cottage cheese
½ cup mango slices (1)
½ cup pear slices (1)
2 dinner rolls (2)
2 tsp margarine
3 graham crackers (1)
Tea or water

Dinner:
3 oz roasted pork
1 cup rice (3)
1 cup veggie stir-fry
2 tsp stir-fry sauce
2 tsp peanut oil
1 cup low-fat yogurt (1)
2 fortune cookies (1)
Tea or water

Snack:
⅓ cup flan custard (1)
4 fresh apricots (1)

2,500 kcal (20 carbs)
Breakfast:
1 cup low-fat yogurt (1)
¾ cup boysenberries (1)
¼ cup granola (1)
½ cup pineapple juice (1)
Coffee or tea

Lunch:
1 cup cottage cheese
½ cup mango slices (1)
½ cup pear slices (1)
2 tsp margarine
3 graham crackers (1)
½ cup vegetable juice
Tea or water

Dinner:
4 oz roasted pork
1 cup rice (3)
1 cup veggie stir-fry
6 a mond nuts
2 tsp stir-fry sauce
2 tsp peanut oil
2 cup low-fat yogurt (2)
2 fortune cookies (2)
Tea or water

Snacks:
⅓ cup flan custard (1)
4 fresh apricots (1)

½ cup fruit sorbet (1)
1¼ cup strawberries (1)

Sample Menu Plan—Day 7

1,200 kcal (9 carbs)

Breakfast:
½ cup egg substitute
½ cup peppers/onions
1 oz low-fat cheese
1 slice wheat toast (1)
1 tsp margarine
2 small plums (1)
8 fl oz skim milk (1)

Lunch:
1 6-inch wheat pita (2)
⅓ cup hummus (1)
2 lettuce leaves
3 tomato slices
1 cup melon (1)
Tea or club soda

Dinner:
½ cup veggie lasagna (1)
1 breadstick (1)
1 cup mix salad greens
¼ cup diced tomatoes
1 Tbsp dressing
17 small green grapes (1)
8 fl oz skim milk (1)

1,500 kcal (12 carbs)

Breakfast:
½ cup egg substitute
½ cup peppers/onions
1 oz low-fat cheese
2 slices wheat toast (2)
2 tsp margarine
2 small plums (1)
8 fl oz skim milk (1)

Lunch:
1 6-inch wheat pita (2)
⅓ cup hummus (1)
2 lettuce leaves
3 tomato slices
1 cup melon (1)
Tea or club soda

Dinner:
½ cup veggie lasagna (1)
1 breadstick (1)
1 cup mix salad greens
¼ cup diced tomatoes
1 Tbsp dressing
17 small green grapes (1)
8 fl oz skim milk (1)

1,800 kcal (14 carbs)

Breakfast:
½ cup egg substitute
½ cup peppers/onions
1 oz low-fat cheese
2 slices wheat toast (2)
2 tsp margarine
2 small plums (1)
8 fl oz skim milk (1)

Lunch:
1 6-inch wheat pita (2)
⅓ cup hummus (1)
2 lettuce leaves
3 tomato slices
1 cup melon (1)
2 small cookies (1)
Tea or club soda

Dinner:
1 cup veggie lasagna (1)
1 breadstick (1)
1 cup mix salad greens
¼ cup diced tomatoes
1 Tbsp dressing
17 small green grapes (1)
8 fl oz skim milk (1)

Snack:
1 cup low-fat yogurt (1)
¼ cup granola (1)

2,000 kcal (16 carbs)

Breakfast:
½ cup egg substitute
½ cup peppers/onions
1 oz low-fat cheese
2 slices wheat toast (2)
2 tsp margarine
2 small plums (1)
8 fl oz skim milk (1)

Lunch:
1 6-inch wheat pita (2)
⅓ cup hummus (1)
2 lettuce leaves
3 tomato slices
1 cup melon (1)
2 small cookies (1)
Tea or club soda

Dinner:
1 cup veggie lasagna (1)
1 breadstick (1)
1 cup mix salad greens
¼ cup diced tomatoes
1 Tbsp dressing
17 small green grapes (1)
8 fl oz skim milk (1)

Snack:
1 cup low-fat yogurt (1)
¼ cup granola (1)

2,500 kcal (20 carbs)

Breakfast:
½ cup egg substitute
½ cup peppers/onions
1 oz low-fat cheese
2 slices wheat toast (2)
2 tsp margarine
2 small plums (1)
8 fl oz skim milk (1)

Lunch:
1 6-inch wheat pita (2)
⅔ cup hummus (2)
3 lettuce leaves
3 tomato slices
1 cup melon (1)
2 small cookies (1)
Tea or club soda

Dinner:
1½ cup veggie lasagna (3)
1 breadstick (1)
1 cup mix salad greens
¼ cup diced tomatoes
1 Tbsp dressing
17 small green grapes (1)
8 fl oz skim milk (1)

Snacks:
1 cup low-fat yogurt (1)
¼ cup granola (1)

1 oz string cheese
24 fresh cherries (2)

Food Distribution for Sample Menus—
Shown for Exchanges and Carbohydrate Counting

Calories	Total Daily Carbohydrate Servings	Carbohydrate Distribution		Total Exchanges
		Meal	Servings	
1,200	10	Breakfast	3	4–5 starches
				2–3 fruits
		Lunch	3	2 milks
				1–2 nonstarchy vegetables
		Dinner	4	4 meats
				3 fats
1,500	12	Breakfast	4	7 starches
				3 fruits
		Lunch	4	2 milks
				1–2 nonstarchy vegetables
		Dinner	4	4 meats
				4 fats
1,800	14	Breakfast	4	8–9 starches
				3–4 fruits
		Lunch	5	2–3 milks
				2–3 nonstarchy vegetables
		Dinner	5	6 meats
				4 fats
2,000	16	Breakfast	4	9 starches
				4 fruits
		Lunch	5	3 milks
				3–4 nonstarchy vegetables
		Dinner	5	6 meats
				5 fats
		Snack	2	
2,500	20	Breakfast	4	11 starches
				6 fruits
		Lunch	6	3 milks
				5–6 nonstarchy vegetables
		Dinner	6	8 meats
				7 fats
		Snack	2	
		Snack	2	

More Menu Ideas

If you feel you consistently lack menu ideas, this chapter will help, but so will other resources. You can try the food section of the newspaper, women's magazines that include weeks or months of meals, cookbooks, library books, the internet, your mother, your friends and neighbors, and cooking classes. Additional resources include registered dietitians, your county extension agent, and the public health department. You may even want to start a recipe club or a dinner club.

PART THREE

Key Aspects of Diabetes Care

CHAPTER 6

Using Blood Glucose Records

U se your blood glucose records to help evaluate your entire diabetes care plan, including your food plan. The only way to know how the food you eat affects your diabetes control is to check your blood glucose levels. By doing so you can learn that certain amounts and types of food will make your blood glucose go high and other amounts will keep your blood glucose where you want it. You will also learn, by observing your blood glucose levels, how physical activity affects your blood glucose.

This chapter will help you:

- Review your blood glucose records
- Know why your blood glucose checks are higher or lower than your target goals

SETTING AND MEETING YOUR TARGET GOALS

The first step in meeting your target blood glucose goals is to know what they are. Target goals are usually given as a range of numbers, not a precise number, because it is impossible to always get the same number. A blood glucose value within the target range will be your goal.

Goals for blood glucose checks are given in the table on page 26. These may or may not correspond to your personal target goals. Your goals may be 20 to 40 points higher. Often the target range for a child will be wider due to inconsistencies in food intake and activity. Discuss your target goals with your diabetes care team.

When you know your blood glucose goals, take a moment to write them here, in the following table. Examples of plasma goals are given in the third column.

Goals for Blood Glucose Checks

	Your Goal	Example Goals
Before meals	_____	70–140 mg/dl
Two hours after a meal	_____	<160 mg/dl
At bedtime	_____	100–140 mg/dl

Your diabetes care should be designed so you can reach your goals. If you are not reaching your blood glucose goals, your food, activity, or medication levels can be adjusted so you can meet them. Blood glucose monitoring will help you decide what to adjust, and then can be used to find out whether the change has the impact you want.

When you consider what you might need to change in order to meet your goals, remember that food is not always the problem. Many times you may hear "you just need to eat less." Yes, food does greatly influence your blood glucose levels, but remember to consider your overall balance of food, activity, and insulin. Sometimes it is easier to make a change in your physical activity or diabetes medicine than food. Examples of changes in a treatment plan to improve blood glucose levels include the following:

- *Rearrange food intake.* Rearrange the time you eat the foods you like. For example, eat small meals and snacks throughout the day rather than several large meals. You are not eating less, just rearranging your food so the insulin you make or take can work with the foods you like to eat.

- *Have more regular activity.* Be active five or more days a week. A little activity everyday may improve your blood glucose levels so your food intake and diabetes medicine, if taken, can remain the same.
- *Take or adjust diabetes medication.* A diabetes medication can usually be adjusted to one's typical eating pattern. This may be insulin, or it may be an oral diabetes medicine. Rearranging medication may be easier than rearranging food intake.

DETERMINING HOW OFTEN TO CHECK BLOOD GLUCOSE LEVELS

How often you check your blood glucose level will depend on the type of diabetes you have, how your diabetes is treated, and whether you are meeting your blood glucose goals. It also depends on how often you want to or are able to check your blood glucose.

Those who take three to four injections of insulin a day or use an insulin pump will check their blood glucose most often. This is because they adjust the amount of insulin they take based on their blood glucose levels. Checking usually takes place before each meal, sometimes two hours after a meal, and at bedtime (before a snack, if you have one).

Those who take two injections of insulin a day usually check their blood glucose less frequently, often just before breakfast and dinner, and at bedtime.

Blood glucose checking regimens vary the most for people with type 2 diabetes who do not take insulin. When first diagnosed, it is helpful to know when your blood glucose is most elevated and how your body reacts to its usual food intake, so checking two to four times a day for several weeks is helpful. The times to check are before breakfast, before and two hours after your main meal, and at bedtime (before a snack if you have one). Then, depending on your treatment plan, if your blood glucose levels are nearing your target goals, you may want to do less checking. At this time, many people will check either twice a day at different times on different days, or three to four times a day once or twice a week.

Always consider increasing your frequency of blood glucose checks if you experience a new schedule, different physical activity, an illness, frequent low blood glucose episodes, a diabetes medication change, a new medication, dental work, or surgery.

REVIEWING BLOOD GLUCOSE RECORDS

Do your blood glucose records look like just a jumble of numbers? They may when you first start checking your blood glucose. Don't feel overwhelmed; there is a way to review them that will help you make sense out of all the numbers.

First, keep in mind that you are *looking for patterns*—patterns of highs, lows, and periods within your target range. For example, look at all your fasting blood glucose values. Are they high, low, or in your target range? To help you see a pattern more clearly, take a colored pencil, pen, or marker and color your high values one color and your lows another color. Those in your target range can be left alone or highlighted with another color. Now the pattern should become clear.

Review the rest of your records in the same way by highlighting your high and low values with different colors. Second, for those values out of your target range check your food diary and review your food, activity, and diabetes medication notes. Were there any changes that could have caused a higher or lower blood glucose? Extra food, less activity, and less medication can cause high blood glucose levels. Less food or skipped meals, extra activity, and more medication can cause low-blood-glucose levels.

OTHER FACTORS THAT AFFECT BLOOD GLUCOSE LEVELS

In addition, to food, activity, and diabetes medications there are other reasons why your blood glucose levels may be different than you expect. These include being sick, having an infection, being under stress, or having your menstrual period. Note these situations in your blood glucose monitoring book so you can best interpret your blood glucose checks.

Sick Days and Infections

High blood glucose levels may be the first sign that you are sick or have an infection. The rise in blood glucose is due to hormonal changes, natural reactions of your body to help you feel better and fight an illness or infection.

At these times you may not feel like eating. If you eat less or don't eat, you may think you should stop taking your diabetes medicine. Don't stop taking it. In fact, you may need more. Also you need to keep eating and drinking fluids. It is best to develop a plan for such times before they happen, so discuss this with your dietitian and doctor.

Do call your doctor if you are unable to keep food down or you have ketones in your urine, or at any other times discussed with your doctor.

You can start preparing now for a sick day by gathering foods to have on hand when your appetite is low, or you are having trouble keeping food down. You may want to keep these foods in a special cabinet or a shoe box, along with other instructions from you diabetes care team. Include several sick day menus that you and your dietitian have developed. When you are not feeling well, you don't want to be running to the store or worrying about having something available that you like at these times.

You may wonder about using low-sugar medicines such as low-sugar cough syrups. These medicines can contain sugar alcohols which can cause stomachaches and diarrhea. They may be helpful because they are low in sugar, but be aware of their side effects.

If you can eat, you can follow your basic food plan—just substitute easy to swallow and chew foods, and your "comfort foods" for other foods. You do not need to replace protein and fat; concentrate on replacing carbohydrate choices with others. Examples include cream soup, plain yogurt, mashed potatoes, ice cream, vanilla wafers, unsweetened applesauce, and popsicles. Other foods to keep in your "shoe box" if you don't usually have them on hand include the following. The serving sizes indicate the amount that is one carbohydrate choice (15 grams of carbohydrate).

- Cans or boxes of soup (nonbroth) – ½ cup
- Cans or bottles of regular soda, like ginger ale – ½ cup
- Packages of regular powdered fruit drinks – ½ cup
- Small cans of fruit juice – ½ cup
- Boxes of regular gelatin and pudding – ½ cup
- Plain crackers like saltines or soda crackers – 6 squares
- Packages of tea – with 1 tablespoon of honey or sugar

You can become dehydrated when you are sick because of sweating, vomiting, or diarrhea. Because of this you need to drink or sip liquids when you can. Even a tablespoon of liquid every 10–15 minutes is helpful. Once you can tolerate this amount, have a ½ cup to 1 cup of food or liquid every one to two hours, or one carbohydrate choice for every hour you are awake. If you are following your basic food plan, have sugar-free beverages between meals.

Other Hormones

Certain hormones in the body rise and fall during different stages of life and different emotional and physical states. Often rises in these hormones cause a rise in blood glucose levels. For example, growth hormones in children and pregnancy hormones in women cause elevated blood glucose levels. It is important in both of these instances not to decrease food intake, because adequate nutrition is critical.

Fluctuating hormones and occasional food cravings during menstruation and menopause can also affect blood glucose levels. Careful monitoring can help girls and women determine their patterns so they can adjust their treatment plans. Keeping track of food intake can help one determine if extra food or an increase in hormones is causing a rise in blood glucose.

Rises in hormones during stressful times often result in elevations of blood glucose levels. Situations like a test, presentation, job interview, or family conflicts can cause blood glucose levels to rise.

Note these situations in your diabetes record book so you can understand why you have blood glucose checks above your target range. Then, once you know why your blood glucose is high you can decide if you can change anything to avoid it from happening in the future, and if so, what. You may be able to adjust your food, physical activity, or diabetes medication. There are times in everyone's life that will create stress—and this may affect blood glucose levels. Learning how to reduce stress can be helpful.

Gastroparesis

Gastroparesis is a medical condition that is caused by changes in the nerves that regulate stomach emptying. When this happens the normal timeframe in which food is digested and emptied from the stomach changes. It is difficult to know if stomach emptying will be normal, slow, or really slow. This makes it difficult to anticipate when the blood glucose will go up after a meal and makes it difficult to determine a course of treatment. This condition more frequently occurs in people who have had type 1 diabetes for a long time, but can occur in people with type 2 diabetes.

One of the first treatments for gastroparesis is a modified food intake to improve the emptying. Many people find that six small, low-fat, low-fiber meals are helpful. Some say that foods begin to "back up as the day goes on." If this happens to you, try to limit solid foods to breakfast and lunch, then switch to more liquid food choices the rest of the day. Also, remain upright, don't lie down, for 30–60 minutes after you eat.

In addition to changes in your food plan, a medication may be prescribed. It is usually taken 30 minutes before a meal and at bedtime, and helps speed up gastric emptying.

Additionally, adjusting the type and time insulin is taken can help. The newer rapid-acting insulins may be taken after a meal once the stomach has started to empty. Blood glucose checks will indicate when this is occurring (they will show a rise in blood glucose) then the insulin can be taken. If insulin is taken before a meal, and stomach emptying is delayed, low blood glucose may occur. This may be one of the first indications of gastroparesis.

Other symptoms that you may have gastroparesis include diarrhea, constipation, vomiting, and stomachaches. The treatment of gastroparesis will help relieve you of these symptoms. Be sure to work closely with your dietitian and diabetes care team to help you plan your meals and avoid any further complications.

Nighttime Low Blood Glucose

Nighttime low blood glucose usually happens only in those who take insulin. It occurs around 3:00 A.M. People who experience this may wake up with night sweats or bad dreams. If the symptoms of low blood glucose do not wake them up, they may wake up in the morning with a high blood glucose, causing them to think they need more overnight insulin or need to eat less before they go to bed. (The high blood glucose happens when the liver makes more glucose in response to the low blood glucose; it is a protective response.) This situation may happen during the day also and is referred to as "rebound high blood glucose."

When you wake up with high blood glucose, it is common to think that you might need to eat less at dinner or bedtime, or take more insulin. This is not so. Eating less or taking more insulin can cause the nighttime blood glucose to go even lower.

To determine if you have nighttime low blood glucose, set your alarm for 3:00 A.M., do a blood glucose check, and write it down. If it is low (below 70mg/dl), treat it, then in the morning call someone on your diabetes care team about it. Also, talk to your doctor if your 3:00 A.M. blood glucose is lower than your morning blood glucose, even if the 3:00 A.M. is not below 70 mg/dl.

Early Morning High Blood Glucose

During the early morning from 4:00 A.M. to 8:00 A.M., the body produces certain hormones that depress the activity of insulin. When this happens, blood glucose levels can rise. If your blood glucose is higher in the morning than when you go to bed, and you may not be having a nighttime low blood glucose, you may be experiencing the "dawn phenomenon." How you treat this depends on your overall treatment plan and should be discussed with your diabetes care team. Treatment may include medication that works in the early morning or decreases the amount of glucose your liver makes during the night (Metformin).

Special Food Situations

If you find that your blood glucose checks are occasionally high or low with no apparent explanation, you may want to assess your specific food choices. Slight differences in some foods may affect your blood glucose response. Evaluating specific foods may seem like a lot to think about. For most people starting a diabetes food plan, the focus is on establishing a food plan and keeping the amount of carbohydrate consistent from day to day. Looking at food more closely becomes important as you feel more comfortable with your basic food plan and you have unexplained high and low blood glucose results.

There are a number of food factors that can influence your blood glucose results. They include the total amount of carbohydrate you eat at a meal or snack, the other foods you are eating with it, the type of carbohydrate you are eating, how the carbohydrate was processed or cooked, the amount of fiber and soluble fiber you are consuming, when and to what degree you have been physically active, what your blood glucose level was before you ate, and whether you adjusted your diabetes medicine for that blood glucose level. Use the following guidelines if you want to experiment with different foods to determine their impact on your blood glucose. Your dietitian can help you with this process.

How to Experiment with Food to Determine Its Impact on Your Blood Glucose

1. Keep food, activity, and medication consistent for two to three days. Keep detailed records of what you eat, when and how active you are, and when you take your medications.
2. Make one change in your food intake and continue to keep detailed records as above.
3. Compare your records; note any changes in blood glucose related to the change you made.

Religious or Other Fasts

You may find it necessary to fast at one time or another. This may or may not be difficult for you with your diabetes. It is more of a concern if you take a diabetes medicine, especially insulin. Sometimes a fast can include beverages. Although not ideal, you can drink sweetened beverages instead of the other carbohydrate you might have eaten at your meals.

Surgery

Prior to surgery you may be asked to limit your food intake and discontinue medications. Then, after surgery you may need to limit your food intake, either the total amount of food or the types of food. As part of your surgery preparation, be sure to ask your doctor for specific directions about your food plan and diabetes medicines. If your surgery is planned, your dietitian can help you prepare menus in advance that you will be able to tolerate after your surgery. It will be a relief to know what you can eat, and to have the food or ingredients readily available. Or, if friends and family want to help with meal preparations, your menus can help them.

CHAPTER 7

Staying Active

This chapter will:

- Identify the many benefits of physical activity for people with diabetes
- Provide guidelines for developing a physical activity plan
- Describe how you can avoid low blood glucose when you are active
- List important safety guidelines you should know and do before increasing your activity

BENEFITS OF BEING ACTIVE

The benefits of activity for people with diabetes, especially those with type 2 diabetes, make engaging in physical activity a "must do." In fact, physical activity is considered part of the treatment plan for people with type 2 diabetes because it helps improve blood glucose control, reduces insulin resistance, and can promote weight loss and weight maintenance. It goes hand in hand with your food plan and is a very powerful tool in your diabetes care plan.

Additional benefits of physical activity for everyone with diabetes include:

- Improved fitness, coordination, balance, and flexibility
- Increased energy level
- Reduced stress, anxiety, and depression
- Extended life expectancy
- Improved sleep
- Increased strength and endurance
- Improved quality of life factors and self-image
- More controlled appetite
- Improved bone density
- Decreased risk of heart disease, stroke, and some cancers
- Lower high blood pressure, LDL cholesterol, and triglycerides

DEVELOPING YOUR ACTIVITY PLAN

The following four steps will help you develop your activity plan:

1. *Make a time commitment.* Identify how much time you can devote to physical activity. New guidelines for physical activity recommend a total of 60 minutes of physical activity on most days of the week. The 60 minutes can be broken into two 30-minute sessions, three 20-minute sessions, or a 40-minute and a 20-minute session. These shorter sessions contribute to the many benefits of physical activity just as longer, more strenuous forms of exercise do. If 60 minutes is too much for you as you begin, set a more reasonable goal—one that you can achieve. Many find that a goal of 30 minutes is more reasonable (and helps with blood glucose control).

2. *Select doable activities.* The best activity for your activity plan is one you enjoy doing and will keep doing. Make a list of activities you like so you will always have options for different weather situations, time limits, and motivation levels. Select activities you can do with others as well as ones you can do by yourself.

You can count routine household activities such as gardening, washing the car, doing laundry, dusting, and vacuum cleaning in your total daily activity. Even parking the car further from an entrance so you need to walk further is an "activity" that provides positive benefits. Activities such as driveway basketball, backyard soccer, and playing catch can also be counted.

If you have physical limitations, consider armchair exercises, strength training with light weights, water aerobics, tai chi, and basic yoga. A wide variety of exercise videotapes offer different levels of activity. Often you can check them out from the local library, video store, or community center. Community centers and fitness clubs offer a range of activity classes that may fit your personal needs and offer support for starting and maintaining your activity plan.

If you are a competitive athlete you can continue your level of activity. People with diabetes play and compete in rigorous endurance activities like marathons and distance bike races, and are able to maintain control of their blood glucose levels. There are pro basketball and hockey players and an Olympic gold medalist who have diabetes. They, and other athletes in other sports, are proof that

> ## What do you want included in your activity plan?
>
> Review your day to see where activities can easily and routinely be included. Look for 10-, 15-, 20-, or 30-minute time segments. Identify what activity or activities you can conveniently do. Make a list of activities you enjoy to remind you of your options.

you can excel in a variety of activities. Your diabetes records will help you determine the adjustments that need to be made to accommodate intense physical demands. Patience, vision, and a supportive diabetes care team can help you accomplish your goals.

3. *Determine the kind of structure you need.* Decide if you need a structured activity plan or if you can flexibly accumulate 30–60

minutes of activity most days of the week. A structured plan may involve doing an individual activity at the same time every day, such as attending exercise classes, or playing an organized sport. Videotapes and regularly scheduled television programs also provide structure. The routine and commitment of a structured activity may help you adhere to it.

4. *Select a time.* The best time to be active is any time that works for you. Lack of time is often given as a reason for not being active. Choose activity times that fit your schedule, and be open to spontaneous activity.

AVOIDING LOW BLOOD GLUCOSE

If you are taking insulin or a diabetes pill that helps your pancreas make insulin, such as a sulfonylurea, Glucovance, Prandin, or Starlix (see the table in chapter 2), you *may* experience a low-blood-glucose episode during or after physical activity. Extra blood glucose checks will help you determine if you need to make adjustments in your treatment plan. Most people with type 2 diabetes will not experience a physical activity-induced low blood glucose with moderate activity. However, if you do take one of these medicines, become familiar with the guidelines below and monitor your blood glucose levels just to ensure they are not low.

Also, review chapter 9 on low-blood-glucose episodes so you are familiar with the signs and symptoms of low blood glucose.

During activity your muscles are working harder and need more energy. During the first 5–10 minutes of increased activity, most of your energy needs will come from the glucose stored in your muscles. This stored glucose is called "glycogen." As your activity continues you have less glycogen available and your body turns to other energy sources—glucose from your blood and fatty acids from your fat stores. This energy helps you continue your activity.

After physical activity and you are resting or going about your daily activities, your muscle is busy replacing its glycogen stores. This can occur up to 24 hours after activity and is why some people with diabetes may experience low blood glucose up to 24 hours after activity. Their blood glucose is being used to replenish the muscle's glycogen reserves that were used during activity.

A half-hour of activity can lower your blood glucose level by 30 mg/dl—more for some, less for others. Checking your blood glucose level before and after activity will help you determine the personal effect of activity on your blood glucose levels.

If you find that your blood glucose goes low during or after physical activity you can make simple changes so this doesn't happen. You will generally need to decide if you should eat extra food, decrease your diabetes medication (discuss this with your doctor), or be active at a time when your blood glucose is elevated (but not when your insulin is peaking).

Needing Extra Carbohydrate

Extra carbohydrate may be necessary before, during, or after increased physical activity to prevent low blood glucose. Your blood glucose monitoring will guide you in knowing if and when you need the extra carbohydrate. The following table provides guidelines for those who take insulin or a medication that stimulates insulin production (see pages 23–24). Those with type 2 diabetes who desire to lose weight, however, are looking for ways to decrease calories so adding a snack is not always their first choice. Decreasing diabetes medication is often the first adjustment. If you do not take a diabetes medication, rarely would you experience a low blood glucose and need extra carbohydrate when physically active.

Note that it is common to need less diabetes medication as you lose weight, so be sure you are monitoring your blood glucose levels and keeping in touch with your doctor during a period of weight loss.

General Guidelines to Increase Food Intake for Activity*

Blood Glucose Level	Intensity of Activity	Snack (Grams of Carbohydrate)
Before activity		
Less than 80	No activity until above 80	
80–180	Light	15
	Moderate to high	15–30
180–300		No snack necessary
250 or greater	Check for urine ketones, if present—no activity	
During activity—at 30-minute intervals		
Less than 120	Light to moderate	15
	High	30
After activity—within 15 minutes		
Less than 120		15
After activity—up to 24 hours		
Less than 120		15

*Discuss the guidelines with your diabetes care team.

Activity intensity (shown in the previous table) is a measurement of your heart rate when you are active. Usually you want to be at moderate intensity when active. Any activity, however, is great.

- Light intensity is walking slowly (1–2 miles/hour), bowling, vacuuming, golfing (with an electric cart), and slow swimming; you can easily sing.
- Moderate intensity is walking briskly (3–4 miles/hour) playing table tennis, golfing (with a pull cart), leisurely bicycling; you can carry on a conversation.
- Strenuous intensity is brisk walking uphill, strenuous bicycling, mowing the lawn with a hand mower, vigorous swimming; you have trouble talking.

Your activity snacks can include any food that contains carbohydrate. You may choose to avoid certain foods, such as those that are high in fat, before or during activity. Examples of 15 grams of carbohydrate include ½ cup of juice, 1 medium piece of fruit, 6 soda crackers, 8 animal crackers, or 2 tablespoons of raisins. Other foods you might like are granola bars, pretzels, low-fat crackers and plain cookies, sports drinks, or sports nutrition bars. See appendix F for a list of additional carbohydrate foods and also read food labels to determine how much contains 15 grams of carbohydrate.

Adjusting Your Diabetes Medicine

It can be fairly easy to adjust your insulin before increased activity to avoid low blood glucose. Sometimes, you may even need to adjust an insulin dose after your activity. Your diabetes care team will need to discuss this with you and it is not something you should begin to do by yourself. The general guideline your diabetes team will talk to you about will be something like this: decrease the insulin that is working the most during your activity by 0–50%. Obviously this is a wide range and will depend on the intensity and duration of your activity.

If you take a premixed insulin like a 70/30 or 75/25, it is difficult to adjust your insulin and you will need to choose an activity time when you blood glucose is high, or add an activity snack. Typically, the diabetes pills are not adjusted for activity, but one may be able to do so with some of the newer ones that are available. Only adjust your diabetes medicine after discussing with your doctor what to do.

High blood glucose. Sometimes activity can cause blood glucose levels to go up. This usually happens in someone whose diabetes is not well controlled and is due to low insulin levels—you need more insulin. There is not enough insulin to help the blood glucose get into the muscle cells. The lack of glucose for muscle cells causes the body to start making glucose; the body thinks it needs more blood glucose, when it actually needs more insulin to use the glucose it has. This causes the blood glucose to go even higher. It is best to not increase your physical activity when this is happening because exercise will just make your blood glucose go higher.

The guideline is to not increase your activity if your blood glucose is over 300 mg/dl. However, if your blood glucose is over 250 mg/dl and you have ketones in your urine, do not exercise.

Ketones. Ketones are a sign that your body is breaking down fat for energy. Urine ketones and high blood glucose mean your body is not working smoothly and you should avoid exercising. The only way to know if you have ketones in your urine is to test for them with a special test strip about three inches long. It is dipped into a urine sample and will change colors depending on how many ketones are present (small, moderate, or large). If your blood glucose before activity is greater than 250 mg/dl and you have ketones in your urine, activity should be avoided.

SAFETY GUIDELINES

Before beginning your activity plan, check with your doctor about any health considerations that may affect your activity choices. For example, if you have eye disease related to diabetes you may need to avoid activities that cause pressure changes in the eyes (valsalva maneuvers) such as straining when lifting weights and vigorous bouncing as in jogging and high-impact aerobics. Or, if you have problems with your feet you may need special footwear or need to choose activities that prevent additional problems.

Other safety guidelines are as follows. The list may look long, but you may already be following many of the guidelines. Don't let the list hinder you from reaching your goals and getting all the benefits from activity.

Activity Safety Guidelines

- Always check with your doctor before increasing physical activity.
- If you are over 35 years old, have had type 1 diabetes for more than 15 years, or had type 2 diabetes for more than 10 years, you should have a graded exercise test before beginning.
- Discuss with your doctor which activities are best for you if you have heart, eye, nerve, or kidney conditions.
- If you take insulin or a diabetes pill that helps you make insulin know the signs and symptoms for low blood glucose.
- Start an activity plan slowly; gradually increase your activity time and intensity.
- Check your blood glucose before and after you exercise to be sure you are in a safe blood glucose range; you may need to check blood glucose levels periodically during strenuous or prolonged activity.
- If your blood glucose is 250 mg/dl or higher before an activity and you have ketones in your urine, do not exercise. If you have no ketones in your urine, do not increase your activity if your blood glucose is greater than 300 mg/dl.
- Wear diabetes identification.
- Wear comfortable shoes and cotton socks. Inspect your feet before and after activity for red spots and sores. Let your doctor know immediately if you have any.
- Have access to and drink plenty of water before, during, and after activity.
- Have access to food if you will be active for a long time or in strenuous activity.
- Inform activity partners that you have diabetes and what they can do to help you if your blood glucose goes low and you need assistance. If you will be alone, let someone know where you will be and what you will be doing if low blood glucose is a concern for you.

CHAPTER 8

Losing Weight

I t is estimated that 80–90% of people with type 2 diabetes are overweight. If this includes you, you may have frequently been told to lose weight. While losing weight offers tremendous benefits, it can be difficult and involves a commitment to lifestyle changes—some simple, others more challenging.*

This chapter will help you:

- Identify the many benefits of weight loss
- Set a realistic weight goal
- Know guidelines for starting·and maintaining a weight management program

THE BENEFITS OF WEIGHT LOSS

The benefits of weight loss (even 10 to 20 pounds) are important to your health and to how you feel. They are especially important to

---

*If you are not ready to tackle weight loss right now, do not read this chapter at this time. You can focus on the information in the other chapters. Later, when you are ready to focus on weight loss, you can come back to this chapter. If you decide now is the time, please read on.

overweight people with type 2 diabetes, but also apply to those with type 1 diabetes who are overweight. Weight loss results in improved blood glucose through decreased insulin resistance (type 2 diabetes) and decreased dosage or need for oral medications and/or insulin. Weight loss also decreases risk of heart disease through lowered high blood pressure, lowered LDL ("bad") cholesterol, lowered triglycerides, and increased HDL ("good") cholesterol. In addition, losing weight decreases the risk of a stroke and some forms of cancer, and helps improve quality of life by improving flexibility, allowing for a wider range of activities and increasing life expectancy.

Also, if you have type 2 diabetes, when insulin resistance decreases, your pancreas doesn't need to work as hard to produce insulin. Smaller amounts of insulin are able to control your blood glucose more easily when you lose some weight. So your pancreas's ability to make insulin will last longer.

Your Personal Benefits

Make a list of all the ways you could benefit from weight loss. Include personal reasons not listed above.

Should You Lose Weight?

The gold standard for identifying whether you should lose weight is the Body Mass Index measurement (BMI). Weight loss is recommended for people who are:

- Obese (BMI greater than or equal to 30)
- Overweight (BMI of 25–29.9) and have two or more of the following risk factors:
  - High blood glucose (diabetes or impaired fasting glucose)
  - High blood pressure (hypertension)
  - High LDL ("bad") cholesterol
  - High triglycerides
  - Low HDL ("good") cholesterol
  - Family history of premature heart disease

- Low physical activity
- Cigarette smoking
- Overweight and have a high waist measurement (over 35 inches for women and over 40 inches for men). By contrast, if someone is overweight and does not have a high waist measurement, or any of the above risk factors, maintenance of their current weight is probably a satisfactory goal.

To figure out your BMI, use the following table. Find your height in the far left column, and then move across that line and find your current weight. Follow that column to the top with the BMI values; that will be your BMI.

Body Mass Index Table

BMI	Normal						Overweight					Obese		Extreme Obesity		
	19	20	21	22	23	24	25	26	27	28	29	30	35	40	45	50
Height	Body Weight in Pounds (weight without clothes)															
4'10"	91	96	100	105	110	115	119	124	129	134	138	143	167	191	215	239
4'11"	94	99	104	109	114	119	124	128	133	138	143	148	173	198	222	247
5'	97	102	107	112	118	123	128	133	138	143	148	153	179	204	230	255
5'1"	100	106	111	116	122	127	132	137	143	148	153	158	185	211	238	264
5'2"	104	109	115	120	126	131	136	142	147	153	158	164	191	218	246	273
5'3"	107	113	118	124	130	135	141	146	152	158	163	169	197	225	254	282
5'4"	110	116	122	128	134	140	145	151	157	163	169	174	204	232	262	291
5'5"	114	120	126	132	138	144	150	156	162	168	174	180	210	240	270	300
5'6"	118	124	130	136	142	148	155	161	167	173	179	186	216	247	278	309
5'7"	121	127	134	140	146	153	159	166	172	178	185	191	223	255	287	319
5'8"	125	131	138	144	151	158	164	171	177	184	190	197	230	262	295	328
5'9"	128	135	142	149	155	162	169	176	182	189	196	203	236	270	304	338
5'10"	132	139	146	153	160	167	174	181	188	195	202	207	243	278	313	348
5'11"	136	143	150	157	165	172	179	186	193	200	208	215	250	286	322	358
6'	140	147	154	162	169	177	184	191	199	206	213	221	258	294	331	368
6'1"	144	151	159	166	174	182	189	197	204	212	219	227	265	302	340	378
6'2"	148	155	163	171	179	186	194	202	210	218	225	233	272	311	350	389
6'3"	152	160	168	176	184	192	200	208	216	224	232	240	279	319	359	399
6'4"	156	164	172	180	189	197	205	213	221	230	238	246	287	328	369	410

Apples and Pears

Interestingly, where you carry your extra weight has an impact on your health. Two shapes, apples and pears, are commonly used to describe the location of extra body fat on men and women. A body that is pear-shaped would resemble a typical hourglass shape with hips larger than the waist. An apple-shaped person carries excess weight in their stomach area.

An apple shape is a sign that a person might have insulin resistance (see definition on page 22). For apple-shaped persons with diabetes, reducing the amount of fat in the stomach area can improve insulin resistance and diabetes control.

DEVELOPING YOUR WEIGHT MANAGEMENT PLAN

The following five steps will help you develop your weight management plan.

1. *Make a weight goal commitment.* Set a realistic weight goal, one that you can achieve and sustain. If you try to lose too much weight too fast, you will probably not be successful. Set yourself up for success.

2. *Select a food plan.* There are a variety of food plans that can help you lose weight. You can count calories, exchanges, or fat grams. Or, you may find that just eliminating unplanned snacking and second helpings will give you steady weight loss.

    Choose a plan that incorporates your favorite foods, allows you flexibility, and offers a range of food choices. Chapter 4 reviews a variety of food plans. Your plan should not feel like a rigid "diet" but rather a way of eating that flows with your lifestyle while helping you meet your weight, nutrition, and diabetes goals.

3. *Determine the kind of structure you need.* Structure in a weight loss plan may be eating precise amounts of foods, eating at the same time and place, keeping detailed records of what you eat, and participating in regular support groups. A precise food plan

with few food choices may help you get started, but may be too confining and rigid in the long term. A less structured plan might give you more flexibility and success that you can sustain. You may find it helpful to switch back and forth between a very structured plan and a less structured plan. Do keep in mind that research shows that keeping a food diary is one of the most effective ways to lose weight and maintain the loss.

4. *Follow a plan for physical activity.* Activity makes losing weight easier. See chapter 7 for suggestions, diabetes activity guidelines, and a list of benefits of physical activity. Regular physical activity is a necessary part of any weight management plan.

5. *Develop a support team.* Losing weight is often easier if you have support from a person or a group, or both. You may obtain different kinds of support for different aspects of losing weight, such as meal planning and education, lifestyle change, and motivation. Do not hesitate to include a support person or group as part of your weight management plan.

Before beginning a weight loss program, check with your doctor about any health considerations that may affect your program. For example, if you have a heart condition you may need special tests before starting a program. Most likely there will be no restrictions, but it is advisable to discuss your plans and goals with your medical team.

Also, if you take a diabetes medication, your doctor may want to decrease the amount you take before you begin your program, or keep in close contact so the medication can be reduced as you begin to lose weight.

SETTING WEIGHT GOALS

Many people are overzealous when setting weight loss goals and this ends up sabotaging their efforts. Be realistic and set a goal that you can both attain and sustain. Then, once you can sustain that weight, reevaluate your situation and decide if and when you want to lose more weight. Bear in mind that losing a large amount of weight may take a long time—one or two years, maybe more. It will be important for you to set many intermediate goals—and celebrate these achievements along the way.

Following are four ways to help you set a weight loss goal. There are others, but not all are as realistic as these and you need to maintain a practical approach to weight loss in order to be successful.

1. *Feel-Right Calculation.* You may choose to lose five or so pounds, then determine how you feel—physically and mentally. Are you comfortable? Do you feel more energetic? Can you easily maintain this loss? If not, work on figuring out ways to maintain the weight loss *before* you try to lose any more weight.
2. *BMI.* Use the BMI chart on page 92 to determine what weight would have you at a BMI of less than 25. If the amount of weight loss needed to reach a BMI of less than 25 seems unreachable, set a more realistic goal that you can achieve and maintain.
3. *10 to 20 Guideline.* Research shows that losing 10 to 20 pounds can have a remarkably positive effect on your blood glucose control. Simply subtract a number from 10 to 20 from your current weight and set that as your goal.
4. *Ten Percent Guideline.* Another easy formula to determine a weight goal is to lose 10% of your current weight. Here are some examples:

If you weigh	180 pounds	lose 18 pounds
If you weigh	200 pounds	lose 20 pounds
If you weigh	250 pounds	lose 25 pounds

DETERMINING YOUR CALORIE NEEDS

The number of calories you need depends on your height and weight as well as your age, body size, physical condition, and physical activity level. Younger adults require more calories than do older adults, and active people require more calories than inactive people.

The best way to determine how many calories you currently eat to maintain your current weight is to keep track of the calories you consume from food and beverages. A food diary, such as the one in chapter 3, can be used to record your food. A dietitian can help you add up your caloric intake, or you can use a calorie book or a computer program.

If you consume about 1,800 calories each day and you maintain your weight, then you need 1,800 calories for weight maintenance. If you want to lose weight, then you need to create a calorie deficit by: (1) eating fewer calories and/or (2) using more calories through physical activity.

Another way to determine your calorie needs is to use the formula in the following table. There are many factors to consider when determining calorie needs which are difficult to include in formulas. However, formulas can serve as a starting point, if you haven't kept a detailed food diary.

Keep in mind that muscles use more calories than fat. Building up your muscles can help you to lose weight faster.

CREATING A CALORIE DEFICIT

We take in calories through the food we eat and use calories through our daily activity. The only way to lose weight is to use more calories than you eat. You can do this by eating fewer calories than you need, or increasing your activity to use more calories, or do both—eat a little less and be a little more active. The goal is to create a calorie deficit so your body uses its stored fat for energy.

The greater the deficit, the faster the weight loss. Yet if you make many changes and lose a great deal of weight, you may not be able to sustain those changes to maintain the weight loss. Consider losing a half-pound to a pound of weight a week as your goal. If you lost weight at this rate for a year you would lose 26 to 52 pounds in a year. Even losing half of that amount would be quite successful.

A deficit of 500 calories a day (3,500 calories a week) will result in

Estimating Daily Calorie Needs for Adults

Step		*Example:* If you want to weigh 150 pounds
1. Determine calories when at rest	10–12 calories per pound of goal weight *Example:* Goal weight × 11 = _____	150 × 11 = 1,650
2. Determine calories for activity	If sedentary, add 30% of calories Line 1 × .30 = _____ If moderately active, add 50% calories Line 1 × .50 = _____ If strenuously active, add 100% calories Line 1 × 1.00 = _____	1,650 × .30 = 495
3. Total rest and activity calories	Add calories from step 1 and 2 _____	1,650 + 495 = 2,145
4. Make calorie adjustments	Add 300 calories per day if pregnant _____ Add 500 calories per day if lactating _____ To gain one pound per week: add 500 calories _____ To lose one pound per week: subtract 500 calories _____ TOTAL calories per day _____	2,145 – 500 = 1,645*

*This number of calories is a starting point for someone who wants to weigh 150 pounds, is a sedentary person (light activity), and wants to lose 1 pound per week.

a 1-pound weight loss every week. You can achieve this deficit in numerous ways, such as:

- Each day: consume 100 fewer calories and increase activity to use 400 more calories
- Each day: consume 250 fewer calories and increase activity to use 250 more calories
- Each week: consume 200 fewer calories a day, and four days a week increase activity to use 525 more calories

Here are a few ways to eat fewer calories:

100 calories fewer: Drink 1 cup of water instead of 1 cup of juice

100 calories fewer: Replace one tablespoon of mayonnaise-type sauce on sandwiches with spicy mustard

150 calories fewer: Choose a single hamburger instead of a double hamburger

150 calories fewer: Drink 12 oz of water or diet soda instead of a 12 oz can of regular sugar soda

200 calories fewer: Have a piece of fruit for a snack rather than a candy bar

200 calories fewer: Eat a small bagel instead of a donut

Here are a few ways to increase activity (approximate calories for a 150-pound person):

200 calories: 1 hour of bowling

250 calories: 1 half-hour of bicycling, 10–12 miles per hour

300 calories: 1 hour of walking, 4 miles per hour

325 calories: 1 hour of mowing the lawn, push-type mower

400 calories: 1 hour of golfing, carrying clubs

400 calories: 1 half-hour swimming laps, freestyle

Easy Calorie Burners

An average day at the office with little walking and no stair climbing might not burn many calories. If you added a 30-minute brisk walk at lunch, you could easily use 150 more calories.

Easy ways to use additional calories throughout the day include:

- Take the stairs instead of an elevator.
- Park the car further from your destination.
- Carry your own groceries.
- Meet a friend for a walk.

- Take several short walk and stretch breaks during the day.
- Do 5- to 10-minute weightlifting sessions with weights or cans of food.
- Lift light weights when talking on the phone.
- Stretch arms, legs, and feet while sitting at your desk, or while reading the newspaper.
- Wash your car by hand instead of using the car wash.
- Use manual gardening tools to mow, trim, and rake.

Other Calorie Burners

In addition to the above calorie burners, look at the following activities and the amount of calories used in an hour. The calories are based on a 150-pound person. A lighter person burns fewer calories and a heavier person burns more.

Calories Burned during Physical Activities

Activity	Calories Burned in an Hour	
	Man	Woman
Light activity Cleaning house Playing baseball Playing golf	300	240
Moderate activity Walking briskly (3.5 miles/hour) Gardening Cycling (5.5 miles/hour) Dancing Playing basketball	460	370
Strenuous activity Jogging (9 minutes/mile) Playing football Swimming	730	580
Very strenuous activity Running (7 minutes/mile) Racquetball Skiing	920	740

Source: National Heart, Lung, and Blood Institute (http://hin.nhlbi.nih.gov).

HOW FAST TO LOSE WEIGHT

The American Dietetic Association recommends losing weight at an average rate of 2–4 pounds per month, or a half-pound to 1 pound per week. If you lose weight faster than this, chances are it will prove difficult to keep off.

If you find, however, that you are losing weight more slowly than this guideline, do not be disappointed. Any slow, steady decline over several months represents success. If you are discouraged, connect with your support team for a review of your plan and all the changes you have made to get where you currently are. They may be able to make suggestions that will help you lose weight more consistently at your desired rate.

Use the above information to set long-term and short-term weight loss goals. For example:

- Long-term goal: lose 8 pounds in 4 months
- Short-term goal: lose 3–4 pounds in 2 months, then reevaluate

You may need to set intermediate goals as well: For example:

- Long-term goal: lose 40 pounds
- Intermediate goal: lose 20 pounds in 9–12 months
- Short-term goal: lose 10 pounds in 4–6 months, then reevaluate

Food plans that promote easy solutions or "miracle weight loss results" may not be safe for someone with diabetes and often do not help with weight maintenance, the most challenging aspect of weight management.

TIPS TO LOSE WEIGHT

It can be fun to set goals and project when you will be at the weight you want to be. The challenge is in resisting food temptations, and keeping track of the calories you eat and the amount of calories you use in a day.

Questions to Help You Set Goals

Think about your weight loss goals. What would you like to weigh? What is a realistic weight for you? Can you attain that weight and sustain it? Pick a realistic weight loss goal. Now set a short-term goal. What do you need to change to attain that? Think of different options that will work well with your diabetes. If you take a diabetes medication, you may need to decrease it when you start to lose weight, so discuss your plans with your diabetes care team.

The following quick tips can help you reach your goals:

- Use less fat all day long. Choose low-fat milk, sour cream, mayonnaise, salad dressings, ricotta, and cottage cheese. Use less margarine, butter, and oil. Avoid fried foods and creamy dishes.
- Avoid high-sugar dessert foods. High-sugar foods such as hard candy, suckers, gelatin, and soda are often available in low-sugar varieties that greatly reduce your calorie and carbohydrate intake. Many sweet, dessert-type foods are also high in fat.
- Do not "super size." Select portion sizes that fit your hunger level and caloric needs. Adding a super-sized soda and fries to a meal can add at least 400 calories and 75 grams of carbohydrate.
- Do not skip meals. If you skip a meal, your body will not work efficiently and you are likely to eat more later in the day. Skipping a meal may also cause a low-blood-sugar episode.
- Add physical activity to your day whenever you can. Adding 10 minutes of brisk activity three times a day will use 200 to 300 calories. If done five days a week, this can result in a 15- to 22-pound weight loss in one year.
- Be mindful of what you eat and drink. Think before you eat or drink. Be aware of and limit snacking, which can easily add 200 to 500 calories a day. Make thoughtful food and beverage choices in restaurants and fast-food eateries, because they offer many high-fat and high-calorie food choices.

TIPS TO MAINTAIN WEIGHT LOSS

The National Weight Control Registry records the stories of people who have lost 30 pounds or more and have kept the weight off for at least a year. Many people have been long-term successes and are part of the registry. The average registrant has lost about 60 pounds and has kept it off for about 5 years. Two-thirds of these successful weight losers were overweight as children, and 60% report a family history of obesity. About 50% of participants lost weight on their own, without any type of formal program. What makes them successful? Here are some of their secrets you may wish to try:

- Keep a daily food diary to track food amounts and calories
- Increase physical activity on at least five days a week
- Walk frequently
- Consume an average of about 1,400 kcal/day (24 percent calories from fat) and expend about 400 kcal/day in physical activity

CHAPTER 9

Preventing Low Blood Glucose

M any people with diabetes are concerned about having a low-blood-glucose episode. A low-blood-glucose episode is typically defined as a blood glucose level below 70 mg/dl. Because your food choices influence your blood glucose levels, and food is used to treat a low-blood-glucose episode, a whole chapter is devoted to this topic.

How will you know if your blood glucose is too low? What will you do? These are questions you will need to answer if you take certain diabetes medications. Those who take insulin are most likely to experience low-blood-sugar episodes; those with type 1 are more likely than those with type 2. Low-blood-sugar episodes are less common if you have type 2 diabetes and take one of the diabetes medicines that help your pancreas make more insulin—sulfony-lureas, Glucovance, Prandin, and Starlix. Additional diabetes medicines may be added to this list as new ones become available. Be sure to check with your diabetes care team to know if the medicine you take might cause a low-blood-glucose episode.

You may, however, take one of these medicines and never have a low-blood-glucose episode. The more tightly controlled one's blood glucose levels are when taking insulin, the more likely a low-blood-glucose episode will occur, at least occasionally.

Other names for low blood glucose include hypoglycemia, low-blood-glucose reaction, low blood sugar, insulin reaction, and insulin shock.

This chapter will help you:

• Learn the signs and symptoms of low-blood-glucose
• Know how to treat a low-blood-glucose episode
• Learn how to prevent low-blood-glucose episodes

CAUSES, SIGNS, AND SYMPTOMS OF LOW BLOOD GLUCOSE

If a low-blood-glucose episode occurs, it is generally easy to treat, and within a short amount of time you can resume your normal activities. The causes of low blood glucose are usually related to changes in your food intake, activity, or medication.

Causes of Low Blood Glucose

Related to food/eating
• Did not eat enough food
• Skipped or delayed a meal or snack
• Had alcohol without food
• Lost weight and didn't decrease diabetes medicine dosage
• Have gastroparesis (delayed emptying of the stomach)

Related to activity
• Increased physical activity more than usual
• Had more intense activity than usual

Related to diabetes medication
• Took too much diabetes medication
• Took diabetes medication too early or too late
• Took other medications that had side effects

Other medicines you may take for different medical conditions may also cause low blood glucose. When you begin to take a new medicine, ask your pharmacist or others on your diabetes care team if it might lower your blood glucose. You can check your blood glucose more often to see if it does.

When your blood glucose level drops below 70 mg/dl, the brain is not getting enough sugar to keep your body active and alert. This causes a variety of feelings and reactions that you and others may notice, such as sweating, confusion, and slurred speech. Not everyone has the same symptoms. The following table lists common signs and symptoms of low blood glucose.

Signs and Symptoms of Low Blood Glucose

Type	Glucose Level	Grams of Carbohydrate for Treatment	Symptoms*	Signs That Others May See*
Mild	50–70 mg/dl	15	Anxious	Anxiety
			Dizzy/light-headed/shaky	Wobbly/poor balance
			Fast pulse	
			Hungry	
			Nauseous	
			Nervous	Nervous mannerisms
			Sweaty	Perspiration; cold, clammy skin
			Tingling lips/mouth	
Moderate	40–50 mg/dl	20	Blurred vision	Difficulty reading or seeing
			Confusion	Inability to talk logically; inability to solve problems

(continued)

Signs and Symptoms of Low Blood Glucose *(continued)*

Type	Grams of Glucose Level	Carbohydrate for Treatment	Signs That Symptoms	Others May See
Moderate			Drowsiness	Sleepiness
			Headaches	Rubbing of temples
			Lack of coordination; delayed reflexes	Poor physical coordination; slurred speech; staggered gait; poor hand-eye coordination
			Mood changes: irritability, anger, sadness, impatience, giddiness	Inappropriate or unexpected mood changes: unusual stubbornness, anger, silliness, crying, pessimistic attitude, impatience
			Nightmares	Tossing or turning during sleep; crying out during sleep
			Stupor	Trancelike (spacey) look; glassy-eyed look
Severe	Below 40 mg/dl	30	Convulsions	Seizures
			Delirium	Irrational behavior, not oriented to time or place; wandering gait, inability to talk clearly
			Fainting (passing out)	Unconsciousness

*You will not have all of these symptoms or signs. Circle the ones you know relate to you.
Source: Adapted from Gehling, E. *The Family and Friends' Guide to Diabetes.* John Wiley & Sons, Inc., New York, 2000.

If hypoglycemia is untreated, your blood glucose level will continue to go lower and you will not be able to think or remember clearly. If you are driving a car, caring for young children, or living alone, the situation could be life threatening. You can avoid these situations by either preventing a low-blood-glucose reaction from happening or treating it quickly when it does happen. Some people make it a habit to check their blood glucose before driving or operating heavy equipment. If in doubt, check your blood glucose and discuss with your diabetes care team what is a safe blood glucose level for you in these situations; usually two consecutive blood glucose checks over 80 mg/dl are recommended.

USING THE 15/15 GUIDELINE TO TREAT LOW BLOOD GLUCOSE

The goal of treating low blood glucose is to raise the blood glucose to a safe level: above 70 mg/dl. The treatment of a low-blood-glucose episode is to eat or drink 15 grams of carbohydrate. Fifteen grams of carbohydrate will often raise the blood glucose level 50–75 mg in 15 minutes—this is called the 15/15 guideline.

Keeping records of your episodes will help you and your diabetes care team to figure out the best treatment guidelines for you in different situations. The following reviews common signs and symptoms, and treatment of the three levels of low blood glucose. You may or may not get this detailed when treating your episode(s). Do follow the guidelines that work best for you.

Level 1: Mildly Low—Blood Glucose 50–70 mg/dl

The mild hypoglycemia, or the first stage of a low-blood-glucose episode, occurs when your blood glucose is just starting to get low. Even though it is called "mildly low," you must take it seriously. Being able to recognize your symptoms and being able to quickly treat any low blood glucose is critical.

15/15 Guideline for Treating Low Blood Glucose

1. If you suspect your blood glucose is low, check your blood glucose with a glucose meter, if one is available. If you are feeling quite low and are uneasy about your feelings, skip this step.
2. Eat or drink 15 grams of carbohydrate and wait 15 minutes for this food or beverage to raise your blood glucose. 15 minutes may seem like a long time, but be patient. If you consume more carbohydrate than needed, you will then have a high blood glucose level. Also, overtreating can lead to weight gain.
3. After 15 minutes, check your blood glucose again to be sure it is up—above 70 mg/dl. If not, eat or drink another 15 grams of carbohydrate. Again wait 15 minutes and recheck your blood glucose. When your blood glucose is above 70 go to step 4.
4. If your next meal is more than 1 hour away, eat another 15 grams of carbohydrate to prevent your blood glucose from going low again before you eat your meal.

Signs and Symptoms. Typical symptoms include shakiness, sweats, tingling lips, dry mouth (some call it cotton mouth), difficulty talking, or a tendency to forget words.

You may experience only one or a few of these symptoms. It is important to know how your body first reacts and "signals" you that your blood glucose is low. Sometimes you may be the only one aware of these signs and symptoms, but other times others might notice them first. You may need to ask others to help you identify how you act during a low-blood-glucose episode.

Treatment. At the first sign of low blood glucose, you need to take action, even if you are in a meeting, at a party, in church, on the telephone, or taking a shower. Stop what you are doing and treat the low blood glucose by following the 15/15 guideline in the box opposite.

Level 2: Moderately Low—Blood Glucose 40–50 mg/dl

Your blood glucose may go from mild to moderate hypoglycemia very quickly, depending on the cause of the low blood glucose and the type of diabetes medicine you take. After you have treated the low blood glucose, reflect on your signs and symptoms, and try to remember if you had symptoms of mild hypoglycemia that you may have missed. This will help you to be better prepared when you have another low-blood-glucose episode in the future.

Signs and Symptoms. At this level you will be able to talk to others, but you might not make sense and you may act a bit differently. If you have not yet identified that your sugar is low, others will probably notice and, if they know you have diabetes, should help you get something to eat or drink. This is why it is important to inform others that you may experience low-blood-glucose episodes, and explain what they can do to help you if they are with you when one occurs. Soon, with treatment, you will be back to normal like nothing happened.

Treatment. Follow the basic 15/15 guideline—but choose foods that require little chewing and are easy to swallow. Also, you may find that you need more than 15 grams of carbohydrate at this level; you may want to consume 20 grams.

Level 3: Severe—Blood Glucose Below 40 mg/dl

This low level of blood glucose, hopefully, will not occur or if so, rarely. If it does, it will probably happen to someone with type 1 diabetes who has lost their ability to feel the early signs that their blood glucose is dropping. This is called hypoglycemia unawareness. There are treatment programs that help those with hypoglycemic unawareness avoid such severe episodes.

Signs and Symptoms. This level of blood glucose can result in convulsions or unconsciousness. A blood glucose check should be done if a support person can easily find a meter and knows how to perform the check. It may be best to get someone to help so one person can do the blood glucose check and the other can start feeding you food. Omit the blood glucose check if you are confident that the blood glucose is low and carbohydrate is needed. The blood glucose must be raised.

Treatment. The treatment depends on if you are awake or are unconscious. Others will need to help you, but they must know what to do and they must act quickly to get your blood glucose up.

1. If you are awake and able to swallow, others can give you jelly, honey, a small tube of cake icing, or glucose gel. Any sugar on the gums of the mouth will be absorbed to help start raising the blood glucose. Usually a beverage or anything that requires chewing is not given. You may try to resist their efforts, but they must be persistent. Total carbohydrate intake must be as much as 30 grams of carbohydrate when blood glucose levels are this low.

2. If you are unable to swallow, are not alert, have passed out, or are having convulsions, someone needs to give you an injection of glucagon, and/or call 911. Glucagon is given as an injection, just like insulin, and raises the blood glucose very quickly. A child weighing less than 50 pounds is given 0.5 mg (half a syringe) and an adult is given 1 mg (the whole syringe). The instructions in the glucagon kit will guide the user.

   It is very easy to use and should elevate the blood glucose 20–30 mg/dl very quickly. Food should be given to the patient once he or she is awake and can swallow. If there is no improvement after one injection of glucagon, another injection can be given, but also call 911. The paramedics will usually give glucose intravenously (IV). Note that glucagon may cause nausea and vomiting so the person receiving it should be either sitting up or lying on their side. Discuss the use of glucagon with your physician. He or she may want 911 called immediately once you have been given an injection of glucagon, and not wait until a second is required. Glucagon is usually given to everyone with type 1 diabetes. It requires a prescription. Friends, relatives, roommates, coworkers, and teachers should have access to your glucagon and know how to do the injection. Periodically check the expiration date of your glucagon, or better yet, mark your calendar when it is time to update your prescription.

SELECTING A CARBOHYDRATE TREATMENT

When treating the first or second level of low blood glucose, there are many options of carbohydrate to choose from—almost any food or beverage that contains 15 grams of carbohydrate. The following is a short list of foods containing 15 grams of carbohydrate. Any 15 grams of carbohydrate food or beverage should raise the blood glucose level about 50 mg/dl in 15 minutes, unless the food is high in fat. Fat can delay a blood glucose increase, so foods such as chocolate, peanut butter on crackers, or milkshakes are usually not recommended.

You may find that a certain food or beverage makes you feel better sooner than another. Or, you may find that with some treatments you need to eat more than with other treatments. This is your personal response, and it is wise to make note of it. You may also find that if you are at level one, you may only need 10 grams of carbohydrate. Again, personal differences and circumstances surrounding the episode influence how your body will react.

Quick List of Foods to Treat Low Blood Glucose

½ cup of fruit juice

½ cup of regular soda pop (not diet)

6 soda crackers

2 tablespoons of raisins

6 Lifesavers

3–4 glucose tablets

1 tube glucose gel

There is no need to add protein, such as cheese or meat, to the carbohydrate treatment. If the protein source is high in fat, it may slow digestion and result in a slower rise in blood glucose, but usually it only contributes additional calories to the treatment.

Examples of Treatment Options for Low Blood Glucose*

If Blood Glucose Is:	50–70 mg/dl: Mild	40–50 mg/dl: Moderate	Less than 40 mg/dl: Severe[†]
Amount of carbohydrate recommended for treatment:	15 grams	20 grams	30 grams
Apple or orange juice	½ cup (4 oz)	⅔ cup (6 oz)	1 cup (8 oz)
Milk	1¼ cup (10 oz)	1¾ cup (14 oz)	2½ cup (20 oz)
Lifesavers, 1 piece per serving, all flavors (3 grams carbohydrate per piece)	5 Lifesavers	7 Lifesavers	
Crackers, saltine-type	6	8	
Sugar, table	4 teaspoons or 4 packets	6 teaspoons or 2 tablespoons or 6 packets	8 teaspoons or 8 packets
Jelly or honey	1 tablespoon	1–2 tablespoons	2 tablespoons
BD glucose tablets (5 grams of carbohydrate per tablet)	3 tablets	4 tablets	
Dex-4 tablets (4 grams of carbohydrate per tablet)	4 tablets	5 tablets	
Glucose gel, 15 grams/tube	1 tube	1⅓ tube	2 tubes

* If you take an alpha-glucosidase inhibitor, such as Precose or Glyset, with a sulfonylurea or insulin, use *glucose*—tablets or gel in a tube—when treating a low blood glucose episode.

[†]Usually food that needs chewing is not given for a severe episode. Sometimes beverages cannot be swallowed. Jelly, honey, and gels may work best. An injection of glucagon may be necessary.

Source: K. Kulkarni, Salt Lake City, Utah, 2002, personal communication.

AVAILABILITY OF TREATMENT

Always have some form of carbohydrate for treatment of low blood glucose available in a purse, pocket, desk drawer, gym bag, backpack, briefcase, or glove compartment. Let others know where this food is kept and tell them how to administer it if needed.

KNOWING WHEN TO TREAT

There are times when you may feel your blood glucose is low, but when you actually do a blood glucose check it is not. You may wonder why you feel this way and whether you should treat these sensations as low blood glucose. It is possible you may be experiencing low-blood-glucose symptoms because your blood glucose has come down fast. In fact, your blood glucose level may be around 150, rather than below 70.

Also, when someone has had high-blood-glucose levels for a long time they find the "feelings" of lower blood glucose different. They may think some of these feelings are low blood glucose, yet they are well above 100.

The best treatment is to monitor your blood glucose every 15–30 minutes until your next meal to see if it is indeed rapidly going low, or getting low enough that a treatment is needed. Eating carbohydrates before they are needed may raise your blood glucose higher than you want. However, you may decide to eat 10–15 grams of carbohydrate because the symptoms are of concern to you. If you do, mark this in your record book and review the circumstances with your dietitian or other member of your diabetes care team.

AFTER TREATMENT

After treating a low-blood-glucose episode, you will want to be sure your blood glucose does not go too low before your next meal. The general guideline is that if your next planned meal is more than one hour away, then you should eat an additional 15 grams of carbohydrate so your blood glucose does not go low again.

Before your next meal your blood glucose should be in your usual target range. For many people this is between 80 and 120 mg/dl. Because you have had a low-blood-glucose reaction and treated it, your before-meal blood glucose may be higher than usual. It may take half a day or a full day to get back to your usual blood glucose levels.

PREVENTING LOW BLOOD GLUCOSE

At the start of this chapter, we identified the causes of low blood glucose. Knowing such causes of low blood glucose can help you prevent these episodes. For example, if you are planning to eat less or be more physically active, or if you are losing weight, you may need to reduce your diabetes medication. However, if you have not planned for these types of changes before, the following table will help you to know what adjustments may need to be made to prevent low blood glucose.

Preventing Low Blood Glucose

If This Causes You to Have a Low-Blood-Glucose Episode:	Then Take These Prevention Steps:
Eating less than usual	Reduce diabetes medication or reduce activity; avoid delaying or skipping meals.
Drinking alcohol	Always eat when you are drinking an alcoholic beverage.
Being more physically active	Increase food intake and/or reduce diabetes medication.
Losing weight	Decrease your diabetes medication. You *may* be able to eventually discontinue your medication.
Taking a new medicine	Some nondiabetes medications can lower blood glucose levels or mask the symptoms, such as alpha-blockers and angiotensin-converting enzyme (ACE) inhibitors for high blood pressure. Check with your doctor or pharmacist before taking any medication.

PART FOUR

Knowing What's in Food

Mastering Carbohydrates

Have you ever wondered how much carbohydrate you should be eating? Or do you wonder if some carbohydrates are better choices than others? This chapter will help you answer these questions. Because so many issues for persons with diabetes center around carbohydrates, this chapter is rather long. Other chapters in this book also address carbohydrates—how much to have in different situations and how they affect your blood glucose at different times (see especially chapters 4 and 14). Feel free to skip around and find the information that you are looking for right now.

This chapter will:

- Identify sources of different kinds of carbohydrates
- Explain the role of carbohydrates in a diabetes meal plan
- Provide recommendations for choosing carbohydrate foods
- Review the glycemic index

WHAT YOU SHOULD KNOW ABOUT CARBOHYDRATES

Carbohydrate is the part of food that affects your blood glucose level the most. All carbohydrates contain sugar, yet we call some carbohydrates "sugar" and others "starches." "Sugars" are short chains of sugar molecules, and starches are longer chains of sugar molecules.

Carbohydrates are found primarily in plant foods like grains, fruits, and vegetables. They are also found in dairy foods like milk, yogurt, sugar beets and sugar cane, and maple syrup. Any food made with these ingredients—such as bread, cereal, pasta, some casseroles and soups, and desserts—is typically high in carbohydrate. For a more complete list, refer to the exchange lists in appendix D; all foods in the starch, fruit, milk, and "sweets, desserts, and other carbohydrates" lists are carbohydrate foods.

Some important points to know about carbohydrate and diabetes are:

- *You can have sugar.* Carbohydrates are broken down very quickly once you consume them. Both sugars and starches end up as glucose in about the same amount of time. That is why you can include sugar in your food plan—because sugar affects your blood glucose in a similar way as starch.
- *Foods containing sugar (table sugar) are usually low in nutritional value.* Any carbohydrate can be a part of your diabetes food plan, but just like people without diabetes, the nutritional quality of your food choices needs to be considered. It is difficult, if not impossible, to be nutritionally healthy if you eat large quantities of sugary foods such as candy bars and regular soda pop. Even the addition of a multivitamin tablet cannot compensate for the nutritious foods you are missing.
- *Keep your carbohydrate intake consistent.* Because carbohydrate foods raise your blood glucose level, monitor the amount you eat and keep it fairly consistent from day to day.
- *Higher-fiber carbohydrate foods offer special blends of nutrients.* Carbohydrates with the most fiber, such as whole grains, fruits, and vegetables, usually contain the healthiest nutrients. The positive health benefits of higher-fiber foods may be due to the unique

combination of nutrients found in these foods. The value of these nutrients—antioxidants, phytochemicals, stanols, fibers, phytoestrogens, and others—are just starting to be recognized and researched. This special blend of nutrients is not found in nutritional supplements or designer foods.

HOW MUCH CARBOHYDRATE TO EAT

When diabetes was first identified, it was known as an illness that resulted in sweet urine. Because of this, diets recommended to persons with diabetes were very low in carbohydrate. In 1922, Leonard Thompson was the first person to receive insulin. He was prescribed a diet with only 20% of its calories from carbohydrate. Today, nutrition guidelines suggest at least double that amount of carbohydrate intake, often from 45% to 65% of total calories.

You can use your typical eating pattern to determine how much carbohydrate should be in your diabetes food plan. The easiest food plan to follow is one that matches your typical eating pattern as much as possible. Rather than trying to fit into a "new" food plan, use your usual eating habits to establish your plan.

By reviewing your food records and your blood glucose records you will be able to tell if any changes in your carbohydrate intake need to be made. For example, if your blood glucose is always high after breakfast, your breakfast may contain too much carbohydrate. However, you may want to continue to keep eating that amount of carbohydrate. Obviously, something needs to change in order to improve your blood glucose after breakfast—and you do have choices.

Your choices to improve your blood glucose control involve food, physical activity, and insulin. You could eat less, be more active in the morning, or take or increase your current diabetes medication that works in the morning. Chapters 6 and 14 provide more guidelines about these types of choices.

Total Carbohydrate

The menus in chapter 5 are ones that many people will feel comfortable following, and are based on 50% of calories from carbohydrate. The following table lists the number of carbohydrate servings at different calorie levels for four different carbohydrate percentage levels. For example, if your calorie intake is 1,500 calories a day and you wanted 50% of your calories from carbohydrate, you would have 12 servings of carbohydrate a day. Each serving of carbohydrate has 15 grams of carbohydrate, which is about how much carbohydrate is in one slice of bread, ½ cup of potatoes, one cup of milk, or a small piece of fresh fruit.

Servings of Carbohydrate (15 grams per serving) for Various Calorie Levels and Percentage of Total Calories

| | Servings of Carbohydrates | | | | |
Carbohydrate	1,200 Calories per Day	1,500 Calories per Day	1,800 Calories per Day	2,000 Calories per Day	2,500 Calories per Day
45%	9	11	13	15	19
50%	10	12	14	16	20
60%	12	15	18	20	25
65%	13	16	19	22	27

Carbohydrate Distribution

Usually the carbohydrate servings are the most important to consider when planning meals, because carbohydrate affects your blood glucose level. Keeping the number of carbohydrate servings the same at each meal from day to day is often a goal of a diabetes food plan. Moving fat or protein from meal to meal usually will not affect your blood glucose level.

Individualizing Your Carbohydrate Distribution

To highlight the point that food plans can be individualized to one's eating preferences, the following table shows seven different ways to distribute carbohydrate in a 1,500-calorie food plan. The numbers in the table relate to servings of carbohydrate. There is no best or correct carbohydrate distribution that is right for everyone with diabetes. Your "best" distribution is the one that fits your typical eating pattern and helps control your blood glucose.

The 1,500-calorie menus in chapter 5 follow the first distribution—four carbohydrate servings at each meal. This may or may not be the "best" distribution for you, so feel free to redistribute the carbohydrate servings if you use these menus.

Some of the Ways 12 Servings of Carbohydrate Can Be Distributed in a 1,500-Calorie Food Plan*

	Servings of Carbohydrate						
Breakfast	4	3	4	4	2	3	—
Morning snack					2		3
Lunch	4	4	5	3	2	4	3
Afternoon snack					2		
Supper	4	5	3	5	4	4	4
Evening snack						1	2

*Based on 50% of total calories coming from carbohydrate, with 12 carbohydrate servings each day.

Adjusting Your Carbohydrate Distribution

If you find that your blood glucose is consistently too high with your usual carbohydrate intake pattern, you may need to make a change in your carbohydrate amount, your carbohydrate distribution, your activity levels, or your diabetes medication. Chapters 6 and 14 will guide you further in making adjustments based on your blood glucose checks.

Often altering the time at which you eat your carbohydrate foods can be effective. For some, eating less carbohydrate at night and more in the morning will help them achieve blood glucose control. Others may need less carbohydrate in the morning and more at lunch. If you have type 2 diabetes, a frequent recommendation is to space your meals four to five hours apart. This allows your body to be ready to make more insulin for your next rise in blood glucose. There are many ways to distribute your carbohydrate servings. If adjusting your carbohydrate distribution and maintaining an activity plan are not able to help you reach your target blood glucose goals, then it may be time to talk to your doctor about taking a diabetes medication.

Low Carbohydrate Intake

Along with the discussion about how much carbohydrate to eat is the issue of low carbohydrate intake promoted by some popular diets. You may be enticed to radically reduce your carbohydrate intake. These diets propose that because carbohydrate raises blood glucose levels, which in turn requires the body to need more insulin, less carbohydrate is better. On one hand, this makes sense. But there are other factors to consider.

Consider what food you would eat if you were on a low-carbohydrate-intake diet. Where would your calories come from? Your choices would be protein, fat, or alcohol. It is easy to understand that alcohol calories are not the answer to replace carbohydrate calories. Neither are high amounts of protein and fat.

Heart disease is the leading cause of death for persons with diabetes. Choosing high amounts of protein and fat typically increases your consumption of saturated fat and cholesterol and increases your risk of heart disease. This is not the answer to high blood glucose levels if your risk for other health complications increases.

The answer includes eating a variety of foods, keeping your carbohydrate intake consistent from day to day and meal to meal, having regular physical activity, and, when needed, using a diabetes medication to reach your blood glucose goals.

If you do want to reduce your carbohydrate intake, consider a reduction to 40–45% of your calories rather than 50–65%. The National Academy of Sciences recommends at least 130 grams of carbohydrate (9 servings) a day (more for pregnant women). Still, be consistent with your intake, have regular activity, and take a diabetes medication, if prescribed. Your dietitian can help you adjust your carbohydrate intake so it fits the eating pattern and the carbohydrate level you want.

THE ROLE OF CARBOHYDRATES IN YOUR FOOD PLAN

Carbohydrate foods provide you with calories and valuable nutrients that are essential for your body to function properly. Most carbohydrates (sugar and starches) are broken down into singular units of glucose. This glucose is used for immediate energy needs, stored as glycogen in the liver and muscle for future energy needs, or stored as adipose tissue (fat).

Differences in Carbohydrates

Research has tested the rise in blood glucose after eating similar amounts of carbohydrate from table sugar, potatoes, and bread, and has confirmed that they all raise blood glucose about the same amount. That research is the basis for the saying that "a carbohydrate is a carbohydrate" when it comes to raising your blood glucose.

This saying is important because people with diabetes can eat sugars and sweet foods and still maintain blood glucose control. For many years diabetic food plans listed sugar and sweet foods as forbidden foods. This is no longer true: sugar carbohydrates can be calculated into the food plan in the same way as starch carbohydrates.

This saying, however, fails to highlight that not all carbohydrates are nutritionally the same. The value of whole grains, fruits, and vegetables in contributing to overall health and preventing certain diseases has already been stated. An easy method for selecting carbohydrates is to choose most often those that contain fiber. This may not always be possible, but it is a useful guideline to help you be selective in choosing your carbohydrate foods.

Calories

Most carbohydrates give you 4 calories per gram. This is fewer calories per gram than you get from fat, making carbohydrates a low-calorie choice when you are on a weight loss or weight maintenance plan.

You can, however, overconsume carbohydrates and gain weight. Also, if you add fat to your carbohydrate, you are adding many calories, making the carbohydrate food no longer a low-calorie choice. For example, it is easy to add gravy or sauces to potatoes and pasta, and margarine or butter to rolls and bread, but by doing so you are more than doubling the number of calories. Alternative choices include enjoying the natural taste of the food, adding herbs or spices that contain no calories, or using low-fat gravies, spreads, sauces, and dressings.

SUGARS

Common sugars are table sugar, brown sugar, raw sugar, powdered sugar, honey, corn syrup, and molasses. Sugar is often combined with fat to make candy, pastries, and other desserts that have little or no nutritional value. Let's admit it, they often taste good, but they also contribute primarily calories and virtually no vitamins and minerals to our daily intake. However, when sugars are found naturally in foods, they are usually with other substances that offer nutritional benefits. For example, fruit is high in sugar yet contains a variety of vitamins, minerals, and fiber. If you want something sweet try fresh, frozen, dried, or canned fruit for a tasty treat. Let's look more closely at the different types of sugars.

Monosaccharides

The simplest sugars structurally are glucose, fructose, and galactose. They are called monosaccharides (one sugar). Glucose and fructose are found naturally in fruits and vegetables. Galactose is part of the sugar found in milk.

Glucose

After digestion most sugars and starches end up as glucose—the glucose that you measure with a blood glucose monitor. Some call this blood sugar monitoring, or say they are measuring their blood sugar. Glucose is the particular sugar that is being measured, so that is why it is becoming more common to use the specific name. Glucose is used throughout this book.

Fructose

Pure fructose raises your blood glucose a little less than other carbohydrates and requires a little less insulin than other sugars for use by the cells. For this reason some specialty food products are sweetened with pure fructose, and you can purchase pure fructose for your own use. The benefit of these foods will depend on the amount of other carbohydrates they contain. It is not necessary to buy such special foods, but if you do, check your blood glucose one to two hours after you eat them to determine whether they benefit you or not. Also, be sure you enjoy their taste; if not, then they are not the best choice for you.

Note that high-fructose corn syrup is used to sweeten many foods and is different than pure fructose. High-fructose corn syrup is not pure fructose. It is similar in composition to table sugar (fructose and glucose), and does not produce the slower and lower rise in blood glucose levels that pure fructose does. Also note that very high intakes of fructose, which are not common (15–20% of total calories), have been shown to raise low-density lipoprotein (LDL) cholesterol and triglyceride levels.

Disaccharides

When two monosaccharides join together, a disaccharide (two sugar) is formed. There are three primary disaccharides in our food.

- *Sucrose* is white table sugar and is the combination of glucose and fructose.
- *Lactose* is found in milk and dairy products and is sometimes called "milk sugar." It is the combination of glucose and galactose.
- *Maltose* is the combination of two glucose molecules.

Other Sugars

There are two other types of sweeteners that are used in foods that are labeled "sugar-free" or "reduced sugar." These are low-calorie sweeteners and sugar alcohols or nondigestible sugars.

Low-Calorie Sweeteners

Low-calorie sweeteners are also called intense sweeteners because their sweetening power is so strong. Small amounts of these sweeteners offer the same sweetening equivalency as larger amounts of caloric sweeteners. Some low-calorie sweeteners are 1,000 times as sweet as regular table sugar.

These sweeteners give you a sweet taste, but no calories or carbohydrate. They may, however, be combined with other ingredients that have calories and carbohydrate. It is necessary to read the nutrition facts panel for total carbohydrate, calories, and fat to determine how these foods fit into your food plan.

Low-calorie sweeteners are listed in the ingredient list on a food label. Some foods will list several low-calorie sweeteners, because blends of several sweeteners can provide a taste that is more similar to table sugar. With blending, less total sweetener is used, as each sweetener enhances the sweetness of the other. The manufacturers choose which sweeteners to blend and can vary the proportions of each sweetener to fit a particular food to give it the best taste. Even some tabletop versions of low-calorie sweeteners are blends.

Tabletop low-calorie sweeteners are very low in calories, and the few calories they may contain are from fillers such as polydextrose and maltodextrin. Because these sweeteners are so sweet, very little needs to be put in a package, so fillers are added to give the product some substance or bulk. The calories the fillers may add do not typically need to be counted as part of one's calorie or carbohydrate intake. Each packet of a low-calorie sweetener has the sweetening equivalency of two teaspoons of table sugar.

Let's review the low-calorie sweeteners that are currently approved for use in the United States and Canada.

1. *Acesulfame Potassium (ace-K)*. Ace-K is about 200 times sweeter than table sugar. It was discovered in Germany and was available throughout Europe before it was brought to the United States and Canada. It is present in a wide range of food products and is typically blended with other low-calorie sweeteners. When it is blended, the resulting sweet taste is quite similar to table sugar. It stays sweet when heated and has a long shelf life.

2. *Aspartame*. Aspartame is about 200 times sweeter than table sugar. It is used in a wide variety of food products but is not without controversy. The American and Canadian Diabetes Associations, as well as other organizations, have confirmed that aspartame is safe. The Centers for Disease Control and Prevention reviewed concerns about aspartame, and found that no symptoms were clearly associated with aspartame. They did conclude that some individuals might have an unusual sensitivity to the sweetener. The Food and Drug Administration (FDA), which approved aspartame, continues to monitor its use and has found no significant evidence of adverse reactions. Aspartame-containing products do have a special warning on the label for people with phenylketonuria (PKU). This is because aspartame is broken down into two amino acids during digestion, and one of these (phenylalanine) needs to be severely limited by persons with PKU.

3. *Saccharin*. Saccharin is 300 times sweeter than table sugar and has been around for over a century, having been discovered in 1879. It was widely used during sugar shortages in World War I and II, before it became popular as a low-calorie sweetener for persons with diabetes. For about 30 years the FDA required a warning label on saccharin-containing foods because of its potential link to bladder cancer. Recently saccharin was cleared of this connection and is no longer considered a risk. Saccharin is blended with aspartame in fountain drinks to help increase the stability of aspartame. In Canada, saccharin is available only as a tabletop sweetener in pharmacies.

4. *Sucralose* (Splenda). Sucralose is 600 times sweeter than table sugar. It is used primarily in beverages and as a tabletop sweetener, but it can be found in a variety of other reduced-calorie foods including ice cream, flavored popcorn, and energy bars. It stays sweet when heated and has a long shelf life. In its granular form it measures and pours like sugar.

The following are other sweeteners of interest.

- *Altiame* is waiting for approval from FDA, although it has been approved in several other countries. It is extremely sweet—2,000 times sweeter than table sugar.
- *Cyclamate* was an early sweetener available for use by persons with diabetes. It is only 30 times as sweet as table sugar but was well liked. In the United States, where it is no longer approved for use due to questions about its safety, it was typically blended with saccharin. It is still approved for use in more than 50 other countries and there is a petition to have it reapproved in the United States. In Canada it can be purchased as a tabletop sweetener and is used as a sweetening additive in medication.
- *Dihydrochalcone* is derived from citrus fruits like oranges and lemons, and is 300–2,000 times sweeter than table sugar, depending on its form. It is said to have a licorice aftertaste. In the United States it is approved for use as a flavoring.
- *Glycyrrhizin* is found in the roots of an Asian and European shrub and is better known as licorice. Interestingly, most licorice candy in the United States is flavored with anise oil, not glycyrrhizin. Glycyrrhizin is 50–100 times as sweet as table sugar. It can be used in the United States as a natural flavoring, but it does not have approval as a low-calorie sweetener. When large amounts of candy and chewing tobacco that contain glycyrrhizin are consumed, headaches, water retention, and high blood pressure have been reported.
- *Steviosida* is a natural sweetener extracted from the leaves of a herb. The name of the herb is stevia, so sometimes the sweetener

is referred to as stevia. It has been used for centuries in Paraguay, and in Japan since the 1970s. It is 300 times as sweet as table sugar. It can be used as a dietary supplement in the United States but no reference to sweetness can be made, because it is not yet approved as a sweetener. Currently the FDA and other worldwide regulating agencies believe that there is insufficient research about how it is metabolized to approve it for use as a sweetener. It is, however, being used by individuals as a sweetener despite its reported slightly anise or licorice taste.

- *Neotame* is 7,000–13,000 times sweeter than table sugar. It is made from amino acids. One of the amino acids is L-phenylalanine, but is not limited for those with PKU. L-phenylalanine is digested differently than the phenylalanine found in aspartame and other foods. It recieved approval for use in the United States in July 2002.
- *Thaumatin* is from a West African fruit and is 2,000–3,000 times as sweet as table sugar. It's reported to have a licorice-like aftertaste. In the United States it is approved as a flavor enhancer, but not as a low-calorie sweetener.

Partly Digested Sugars (Sugar Alcohols)

Some sugars are not completely digested. You may recognize these sugars by the terms "sugar alcohol," "polyols," or "sugar replacers." Because they really do not contain any alcohol, the term "sugar alcohol" is often confusing. However, you will see this term used in the nutrition facts panel of a food label under Total Carbohydrate.

If there is only one sugar alcohol in a food, the specific ingredient name is listed (e.g., sorbitol). If two or more are used, the panel says "sugar alcohol." The individual names are always listed in the ingredient list. They include sorbitol, mannitol, xylitol, isomalt, malitol, lactitol, and hydrogenated starch hydrolysates. You can find these in a variety of foods including candy, cookies, throat lozenges, and chewing gum.

Main Points to Know. There are three main points to know about sugar alcohols:

- They are often found in foods that are labeled "sugar-free" or "no added sugar," but the food may still contain calories from other carbohydrates.
- They may cause stomachaches and excess gas.
- They should not be used to treat hypoglycemia.

We do not have enzymes in our mouth to start the digestion of sugar alcohols, so unlike other caloric sweeteners, sugar alcohols will not cause tooth decay. In fact, since they are not completely digested, they have pluses and minuses. On the positive side, they produce a smaller rise in blood glucose than regular sugar, and give you additional low-carbohydrate food choices. On the negative side, they can cause stomachaches, excess gas, and even diarrhea because they are partially digested. Eating smaller amounts of such foods at one time can help eliminate the problem.

Sugar alcohols are sometimes added to food products that are sweetened with a low-calorie sweetener because they add bulk (filler) and few calories. When you take sugar out of a food, you not only lose the sweet taste, you also lose bulk. The sugar alcohols replace the bulk while the low-calorie sweetener replaces the sweet taste (since sugar alcohols are only half as sweet as other caloric sweeteners).

Additional Points to Know. There are two additional points that those who adjust their before-meal insulin based on the carbohydrate content of the meal should know.

- Sugar alcohols produce a slower and lower rise in blood glucose than other sugars or starches.
- On average, only half of the sugar alcohol carbohydrate needs to be counted into your carbohydrate grams, because only half of it is digested.

Because sugar alcohols are only partially digested, only half the carbohydrate grams listed next to the specific sugar alcohol (e.g., sorbitol) or the general term "sugar alcohol" are available to raise your blood glucose. To get the true amount of available carbohydrate from a food with a sugar alcohol, subtract half of the sugar alcohol grams from the Total Carbohydrate amount. Using the nutrition facts panel in the figure below as an example:

- Divide sorbitol grams by two: $16 \div 2 = 8$.
- Subtract 8 from 19 = 11 grams of total carbohydrate that are available to raise your blood glucose.

For some people, this will be a small amount of carbohydrate and will not make a difference. For others, however, it may help with blood glucose control, and choosing the amount of food to eat.

Nutrition Facts
Serving Size: 2 pieces (40g)
Servings Per Container: About 2
Amount Per Serving
Calories 180
Total Fat 11g
Total Carbohydrate 19g
Sugars 3g
Sorbitol 16g
Protein 4g

Simplified sugar-free candy food label

Lactose

Lactose is an undigestible sugar for people with lactose intolerance, because they lack the enzyme lactase that breaks it down to its one-sugar units (glucose and galactose). When they consume too much lactose at one time they may experience nausea, cramps, bloating, gas, and diarrhea about 30 minutes to 2 hours after consuming lactose. Sometimes small amounts, like that in a fourth of a cup of milk, cause no discomfort whereas a whole cup would be intolerable. Others may be able to consume ice cream and aged cheeses, such as cheddar and Swiss, but not other dairy products. Dietary control of lactose intolerance depends on each person's learning through trial and error how much lactose he or she can handle.

Many preprinted diets for persons with diabetes include milk. This highlights the need to have an individualized food plan. If you eliminate or limit milk products, you may want to see a registered dietitian to ensure you are meeting your nutritional needs. You might want to choose milk products that have the lactose broken down, such as lactose-free milk, acidophilus milk, yogurt, buttermilk, sour cream, and lactose-free cheeses. Or you can purchase the enzyme lactase in liquid form from most drug stores and add it to your milk. Another choice is soy milk fortified with calcium and vitamin D. Some choose to chew a tablet containing the enzyme before meals so they can comfortably eat a variety of lactose-containing foods. Green vegetables such as kale and broccoli are high in calcium, as are fish with edible bones such as sardines and salmon.

If you avoid lactose-containing foods because you are ovo-vegetarian (do not eat meat, milk, or milk products) or vegan (avoid all foods of animal origin), you can still follow a healthy diabetes food plan.

STARCHES

Starches are plant foods or foods made from grains. Examples include bread; crackers; pasta; rice; cous cous; polenta; starchy vegetables such as potatoes, corn, green peas; and dried beans and peas. In many countries, starches are the center of a meal and come in a variety of different tastes, texture, and colors.

Starch carbohydrates are chains of more than three sugar units that are called oligo- or polysacchrides. Enzymes in your mouth start to break down these chains immediately, so the expected rise in blood glucose is often the same as when you eat equal amounts of carbohydrate from sugar.

FIBER

Some parts of some starches cannot be digested or are only partially digested by bacteria in the large intestine. These components are called *dietary fiber*. Dietary fiber is found in foods that have structure or shape, like fruits and vegetables; in whole grains; in seeds like in tomatoes and strawberries; and in dried beans and peas.

It's possible to alter the amount of fiber in a food by how it is processed or how long it is cooked. For example, whole potatoes have more fiber than mashed potatoes, and an apple has more fiber than apple juice. Names for fiber include cellulose, hemicellulose, pectin, beta-glucans, gum, and lignin.

You can purchase fiber supplements that can help with constipation or diarrhea, but they will not offer the same nutritional value you receive from eating the actual foods that contain the fiber. Nutrition scientists are finding that small amounts of other nutrients found with fiber may also help lower your risk of certain diseases, lower your cholesterol levels, and even lower your blood glucose levels. These nutrients include phytochemicals, selenium, tocotrienol (a form or vitamin E), lignans, and soluble fiber.

The value of fiber can easily be seen in the number of health claims that are allowed on food packages that contain fiber. These range from preventing heart disease to preventing certain cancers. See the list of allowed health claims in chapter 16.

How Much Fiber to Eat

The National Academy of Sciences recently set recommendations for total fiber intake. Food labels list the amount of fiber in a food. You can use that information to add up how much fiber you eat, and you can use the table on page 138. The recommendation is based on how many calories you eat. Because men typically eat more calories, they need more fiber. See the following table.

How Much Fiber to Eat Each Day

	Men	Women
50 years and younger	38 grams	25 grams
More than 50 years	30 grams	21 grams

Total fiber intake includes dietary fiber and functional fiber. Functional fiber is a new term. It refers to fiber that is man-made or a fiber that has been extracted from a food. These fibers have been studied and have shown that they have beneficial health effects, such as lowering blood cholesterol or maintaining blood glucose levels.

New products may become available that say they are high in a specific functional fiber. It is important to still consume a good amount of fiber from food.

Two Types of Dietary Fiber

There are two types of dietary fiber: soluble and insoluble. Researchers test fibers to see if they dissolve in water or not. Put simply, if a fiber dissolves then it is soluble; if not, it is insoluble. Most foods that contain fiber contain both types. Both will help you feel full and satisfied after eating.

The nutrition facts panel will list the amount of fiber in a food as dietary fiber. This is the total amount of fiber, including the soluble and insoluble amounts. Some labels will list the amount of soluble fiber separately underneath the amount of dietary fiber.

Fiber intake should be between 20 and 40 grams of total dietary fiber a day. For many, this is an increase in fiber intake, because the average intake is only 12–17 grams of fiber a day with only 3–4 grams of soluble fiber.

1. *Insoluble Fiber.* Insoluble fibers are cellulose, hemicellulose, and lignins. Foods they are found in include wheat, rye, barley, and some vegetables. Foods high in insoluble fiber are often recommended to help digestion or constipation; some call them natural laxatives. Because they do not dissolve in water, they move through the digestive tract as a group of sugar units. As they move they help push other food substances along. Insoluble fiber absorbs water so it bulks up.

2. *Soluble Fiber.* Soluble fibers include pectins, beta-glucans, gums, and mucilages. Pectins are found in apples and citrus fruits, and beta-glucans in oats and barley. Other excellent sources of soluble fiber include dried beans and peas, broccoli, carrots, berries, and prunes. Soluble fiber is important to those with diabetes because it does the following:
   - It reduces cholesterol levels. Soluble fiber forms a gel when mixed with liquids in the body. (Soluble fiber is sometimes called

viscous fiber because it forms a gel and doesn't truly dissolve.) This gel binds with excess cholesterol and removes it from the body; it is excreted, along with other excess nutrients, in the stool. The National Cholesterol Education Program (NCEP) recommends 10–25 grams of soluble fiber a day to help lower cholesterol levels if your LDL cholesterol level is above 100 mg/dl.

• In very high amounts, it can improve blood glucose control. The reason that soluble fiber reduces blood glucose levels is not clearly understood. A recent *New England Journal of Medicine* research study found that 25 grams of soluble fiber [50 grams of dietary (total) fiber] a day improved blood glucose control, improved blood fats levels, and improved insulin resistance.

How to Increase Fiber Intake

General guidelines for increasing fiber intake include choosing more whole grains, fruits, and vegetables as part of your meals (see the following table). Most fruits and vegetables are good sources of fiber. Whole grains include whole wheat, oats, barley, brown rice, bulgur, buckwheat (kasha), corn, millet, and quinoa. The Dietary Guidelines for Americans specifically state that we should eat at least two servings of fruit, three servings of vegetables, and three servings of whole grains each day. These suggestions fit well with a diabetes food plan.

How to Increase Fiber Intake

Instead of These Low-Fiber Foods:	Choose These High-Fiber Foods:
White bread	Whole-grain bread
Processed breakfast cereal	Whole-grain cereals, bran, oatmeal, or cereal with dried fruit
Mashed potatoes	Whole-grain pasta, legumes, baked potato with skin, or sweet potatoes
White rice	Brown rice, wild rice, quinoa, millet, or whole-wheat cous cous
Fruit juices	Fresh, frozen, canned, or dried fruit
Plain crackers, muffins, cookies, or cakes	Items made with whole-grain flour, bran, or oatmeal; dried fruit

Gradually Increase Foods Higher in Fiber

Higher-fiber foods such as whole grains, oats, and dried beans may make you feel bloated or produce excess gas when eaten. The more you eat them, the more you will adjust and the side effects usually decrease over time. These foods offer extra nutrition and health benefits so don't give up on them. Gradually increase your intake and drink extra water to increase their digestibility.

1. *Fruits and Vegetables.* A national campaign, called 5 a Day, encouraging people to eat five to nine servings of fruits and vegetables each day, has raised the awareness of eating fruits and vegetables. Unfortunately, many Americans are not meeting this goal despite research citing the value of fruits and vegetables in preventing and treating many health conditions, including cancer, heart disease, and high blood pressure.

    Although it can be quite easy to consume five servings a day, it may initially require some extra thought about food choices. In the diabetes food plan, fruit is either included as a fruit serving or as a carbohydrate serving, and is often included at two or three meals each day. Fresh, frozen, or canned fruit (water or juice packed, not in heavy syrup) provide more nutrients than fruit juice so try to choose them more often.

    Most nonstarchy vegetables are often considered "free" because they have few calories, and a food plan may include one to two servings at lunch and dinner. Vegetables also make great snacks because they are low in calories and are usually crunchy so they can be a satisfying low-calorie, low-carbohydrate choice. Some vegetables, like potatoes and green peas, are starchy and are counted as starch or carbohydrate choices in the diabetes food plan, similar to fruits. Because of this, count them as either starch or carbohydrate servings in your food plan.

2. *Whole Grains.* On average, we only eat one serving of whole-grain foods a day. Perhaps this is partly due to the difficulty in identifying a whole-grain food. Whole grains contain all three parts of the grain—the bran, the germ, and the endosperm.

The only way to know if a food contains a whole grain is to read the ingredient list. If the grain is wheat, it must read "whole wheat" to be a "whole grain." A bread may be labeled seven-grain, or multi-grain, and be brown in color, but if the ingredient list does not list "whole wheat," it may not be a whole-grain food. However, if the grain used is oats or barley, the word "whole" is not needed. The label can read "oats" or "barley" and the food will be a whole-grain food. Look for foods that list a whole grain first in the ingredient list.

Whole grains have many health benefits. They can help prevent type 2 diabetes, reduce cholesterol levels, reduce blood pressure, improve insulin sensitivity, and improve blood glucose control. For these and other reasons, it is important for those with diabetes and their family members to increase their intake of whole-grain foods.

An easy way to increase your whole-grain intake is to start your day with a whole-grain cereal, then use whole-grain bread in a sandwich at lunch. Another way would be to have whole-grain toast for breakfast, and whole-grain crackers or popcorn for a snack. You can add more whole grains to your evening meal by choosing one or more of the whole grains listed in the previous table or the following table for your evening carbohydrate servings.

How to Increase Whole-Grain Intake

Choose foods that name one of the following ingredients *first* on the label's ingredient list:

Brown rice	Graham flour	Popcorn	Whole rye
Bulgur (cracked wheat)	Oatmeal	Whole grain corn	Whole wheat
	Pearl barley	Whole oats	

Try some of these whole-grain foods: whole-wheat bread, whole-grain ready-to-eat cereal, low-fat whole-wheat crackers, oatmeal, whole-wheat pasta, whole barley in soup, and tabouli salad.

Note: "Wheat flour," "enriched flour," and "degerminated corn meal" are not whole grains.

Source: Dietary Guidelines for Americans, 5th edition. United States Department of Agriculture, United States Department of Health and Human Services, 2000.

Count Grams of Fiber

To reach a certain amount of fiber a day, you can count grams of fiber that are listed on food packages. The following table includes the fiber content of a variety of foods. Most food amounts listed in this table are one serving of carbohydrate and contain about 15 grams of carbohydrate. The "other vegetables," however, contain the least amount of carbohydrate—5 grams in a 1-cup serving when raw—making them a popular choice for increasing total and soluble fiber content.

Comparison of Foods and Their Fiber Amounts

Food	Amount	Dietary (Total) Fiber (grams)	Soluble Fiber (grams)
Bread			
White	1 slice	0.6	0.3
Wheat	1 slice	1.0	0.3
Oatmeal	1 slice	1.1	0.6
Rye	1 slice	1.5	0.8
Cereal			
Rice Krispies	¾ cup	0.2	0.1
Corn Flakes	¾ cup	0.6	0.1
Cream of wheat, quick	½ cup	0.5	0.2
Cream of wheat, regular	½ cup	0.6	0.2
Cheerios	¾ cup	2.2	0.7
Oatmeal, quick	½ cup	2.0	1.0
Oatmeal, regular	½ cup	2.0	1.0
Fruit			
Apple juice	½ cup	0.2	0.0
Apple, with skin	1 medium	3.0	0.8
Banana, fresh	1 small	2.1	0.6
Blackberries	¾ cup	5.7	1.0
Blueberries	¾ cup	2.9	0.3
Orange	1 small	2.3	1.4
Raspberries	1 cup	8.4	0.9
Strawberries	1¼ cup	4.1	1.1
Dried beans			
Kidney, cooked from dried	½ cup	5.7	2.8
Navy, cooked from dried	½ cup	5.8	2.2
Pinto, cooked from dried	½ cup	7.4	1.9
Nonstarchy vegetables			
Broccoli, cooked from frozen	½ cup	2.8	1.4
Broccoli, raw	1 cup	2.6	1.0
Carrots, raw	1 cup	3.3	1.7
Tomato, raw	1 cup	2.0	0.2

Note: Each serving of bread, cereal, fruit, and dried beans contains 15 grams of carbohydrate and is equal to 1 carbohydrate serving. Each serving of nonstarchy vegetables contains 5 grams of carbohydrate and is considered a "free" food in that amount.

Source: Spiller, GA: *CRC Handbook of Dietary Fiber in Human Nutrition, 3rd edition.* CRC Press, Boca Raton, Florida, 2001.

Sample Meals

The following menus suggested by the American Institute of Cancer Research show how a day's worth of meals can easily include two servings of fruit, three servings of vegetables, and three servings of whole grains. The fiber in these three meals totals 27 grams.

- A breakfast that includes a cup of oatmeal (4 grams) and a banana (2 grams)
- A lunch sandwich of two slices of whole-wheat bread (2 grams), filled with a quarter-cup of hummus (4 grams), followed by an orange (2 grams) for dessert
- A dinner that includes a medium baked potato with skin (3 grams), a half-cup of broccoli (3 grams), and a cup of strawberries (4 grams)
- Evening snack of 3 cups popcorn (3 gms), or 1 apple (3 gms)

Adjusting Total Carbohydrate

Fiber grams are part of the total carbohydrate amount listed on a food label. Since fiber is not digested, you can subtract it from the total carbohydrate amount. This is only necessary when you are having 5 grams or more of fiber at a meal. And it may only be necessary for those who are being precise with their carbohydrate intake and adjusting a rapid- or short-acting insulin based on how much carbohydrate they are eating.

Here's an example: If you had the dinner meal listed above with 10 grams of fiber, you would subtract the 10 from the total amount of carbohydrate at that meal (45 grams). Your before-meal insulin dose would be based on the adjusted amount of carbohydrate (35 grams). If you do adjust for fiber, make a note in your record book so you can later assess whether that adjustment worked for you.

Increasing Satiety

If you are trying to lose weight and worry about constantly being hungry, review your food choices. Are you choosing foods high in fiber? A classic study looked at the satiety (feeling of fullness) effect of three forms of apples: apple juice, applesauce, and whole apples. The researchers asked the study participants how full and satisfied they felt after eating each food item. Apples (containing more fiber) were the most satisfying, followed by applesauce and then the low-fiber juice. Use fiber to your advantage when losing and maintaining your weight.

GLYCEMIC INDEX

The glycemic index is a system to categorize carbohydrate foods based on how high they raise the blood glucose level after they are eaten. All foods are compared to either glucose or white bread. The rise in blood glucose after eating glucose or white bread is given a value of 100%. If a food raises the blood glucose level more, the glycemic index of that food will be greater than 100%. If a food gives a lower rise in blood glucose, the glycemic index will be less than 100%.

Glycemic index research studies typically included small groups of people (not all with diabetes) and based the glycemic index value on the average for the group. Some may have had higher or lower responses. Determining your own personal response to foods may be the most valuable to you, especially to those who are being precise with their food intake and adjusting insulin based on a food's glucose excursion (rise in blood glucose after a meal). It may be another piece in the puzzle when trying to figure out why your blood glucose may not be what was expected.

There are, as you might guess, pros and cons to using this method. A positive is that this system provides further guidance in evaluating food records. On the negative side, there are many factors that affect the blood glucose response, making it difficult to expect a precise response every time a certain food is eaten. In fact, when foods are eaten in combinations, the blood glucose response is usually predicted by the *total amount* of carbohydrate, and not individual glycemic index values.

One's response can vary depending on one's blood glucose level before a meal, how the food is processed or prepared, what else is eaten with the food, the amount of food you eat, how quickly the food passes through your digestive tract, the time of day the food is eaten, and possibly your activity and diabetes medication. The rise in blood glucose may also be affected by your blood glucose before the meal.

If a meal is high in fat, it slows the digestion of the meal and rise in blood glucose. Thus, ice cream has a low glycemic index because of its fat content. If a food is processed differently or in a different state than what is evaluated, it can cause a different glycemic response. An unripe banana, for example, will cause a different response than an overripe one. Even growing conditions, such as type of soil and weather, can influence a food's precise carbohydrate content and therefore its glycemic response. Some sugary foods have a low glycemic index because they contain sucrose, which breaks down to glucose and fructose. Fructose causes less of a rise in blood sugar. Consider the nutritional value of foods and not solely their glycemic index if you use this system.

Despite the many factors that can affect the glycemic response to a food, you may want to review the glycemic index charts in appendix H and note the values of some of the foods that you eat. You can use this information when reviewing your blood glucose records. Do you notice a higher blood glucose after you have had a food with a high glycemic index? After observing your reaction to a variety of foods, you may discover that there are some foods that you seem to be more sensitive to than others. If this is so, you can eat smaller amounts of those foods and keep your blood glucose in your target range.

CHAPTER 11

Understanding Protein

P rotein is a nutrient that is found in both plant- and animal-
based foods. Foods that are high in protein are fish, meat,
poultry, milk, cheese, yogurt, nuts, seeds, dried beans and
peas, and soy products such as soymilk, soy nuts, and tofu.

This chapter will:

- Explain what proteins are and what they do
- Explain the role of protein in a diabetes food plan
- Provide recommendations for how much protein to eat

WHAT YOU SHOULD KNOW ABOUT PROTEIN

Protein is primarily used to build and repair body cells and tissues.
An adequate amount of insulin is needed for protein to be used.
When your blood glucose is in control, you have enough insulin;
otherwise some of the functions of protein may be impaired.

Each protein consists of a chain of amino acids. There are 20
amino acids that can be linked up in many different combinations
and patterns to form a variety of different kinds of proteins. The
protein you eat gets broken down to its amino acids very quickly,

and then your body uses them to meet its needs. For example, if you have a sore that is healing, your body will send amino acids to this site to help out. If you have been exercising, your body will send amino acids to your muscles to build more muscle cells.

Proteins form part of every cell in your body—from your hair down to your toes. Proteins make up the enzymes you use to digest food and to make new cells. Other proteins make up the DNA that directs what your body's cells do.

Some important points to remember about protein and diabetes are:

- *Extra protein is stored as fat.* As with other food substances that contain calories, protein can cause weight gain if you consume too much. Americans often eat twice as much protein as they need for maintenance and repair; the excess is primarily stored as body fat.
- *Choose protein sources that are low in saturated fat and cholesterol.* Protein foods can be high in saturated fat and cholesterol. Consider eating one or two low-fat vegetarian meals a week and one to two fish meals a week to help decrease your intake of saturated fat and cholesterol.
- *It is not necessary to have a high-protein food at every meal.* Food plans for diabetes used to always include a high-protein food at every meal and snack. This is not necessary.
- *Have your doctor check your urine for protein.* Small amounts of protein in the urine are a sign that your kidneys are having trouble.

HOW MUCH PROTEIN TO EAT

Many Americans consume high amounts of protein thinking this will help them build muscles and control their weight. This is not so. The body needs a limited amount of protein and stores the excess as body fat. Because of this and the high fat content of many protein foods, keep your protein intake to about 15–20% of your total calories. See the following table to know how many grams this is. New

Amount of Protein at Various Calorie Levels When Protein Is 15–20% of Calories

Daily Calorie Amounts	1,200	1,500	1,800	2,000	2,500
Calories from protein	180–240	220–300	270–360	300–400	375–500
Grams of protein	45–60	56–75	68–90	75–100	94–125

nutrition guidelines give a wider intake range—10–35% of total calories. Your protein intake will depend on how much carbohydrate and fat you eat.

To quickly determine how many grams of protein you have each day, count:

- 2 grams of protein for each serving of pasta, bread, crackers, and starchy vegetables
- Each of these servings as 7 grams; 1 ounce of cooked meat, chicken, and fish; 1 ounce of cheese; ¼ cup cottage cheese, 1 egg, ¼ cup egg substitute, ½ cup tofu
- 7 grams for each ½ cup of cooked beans, peas, and lentils
- 8 grams per one cup of milk or yogurt

Grams of protein are also listed on food labels, so you can use those amounts to help you total your daily protein intake.

There are groups of people who have special protein needs, and may require the higher percentages of protein. These groups include growing children, pregnant women, strength and endurance athletes, and elderly individuals who consume few calories.

Protein Distribution

For blood glucose control, it is not necessary to be as exact with your protein intake as with your carbohydrate intake. If you omit your protein, your blood glucose will usually not be affected. For example, your food plan includes 3 ounces of meat or other protein at lunch which you usually have in a sandwich. You decide to have a vegetarian sandwich of bread and vegetables, instead of your usual meat sandwich. Your blood glucose after your meal should be similar to the days you have the meat sandwich.

On the other hand, there may be times when you eat more protein than usual at a meal. For example, you might have a large omelet for breakfast, an extra serving of turkey on Thanksgiving, or an extra large steak at a steak house restaurant. Usually this will not affect your blood glucose control. Some people who use insulin pumps and monitor their blood glucose levels very carefully find they do not need extra insulin for extra protein. What they do find is that if their high-protein meal is also high in fat, they will have a delayed rise in blood glucose because an increase in fat intake slows digestion.

Some food plans suggest a range of protein servings, such as 0–1 servings at breakfast, 2–4 at lunch, and 3–5 at supper. Those who are on weight-loss plans will want to be more exact with their intake, because extra calories from the extra protein servings can delay or prevent weight loss.

Protein with Every Meal and Snack

It used to be a standard diabetes recommendation to have a complete protein at breakfast (one egg, one slice of cheese) and with all snacks (cheese, meat, peanut butter, etc.). It was thought that the small amount of protein would slow the rise in blood glucose, and would help prevent low blood glucose episodes. In the American Diabetes Association's latest nutrition recommendations it is explained that this suggestion was finally tested and found to be untrue. Meals with and without protein resulted in the same rise in blood glucose. For many, omitting unnecessary protein can help decrease caloric intake and promote weight loss.

Omitting protein from snacks may be a major change in habit and way of thinking for many. If you feel you need the protein, check it out yourself as your body may react differently to protein than the research indicated. Keep your food intake and activity consistent for several days and check your blood glucose before and two hours after the meal or snack you are "testing." Then, eliminate this protein for several days and compare your blood glucose levels. This will be your personal guide for whether or not you need to include protein.

Very High Protein Intakes

High-protein diets for weight loss have regained popularity in recent years. Proponents of high-protein diets make two claims about these diets: first, that very high protein intakes are not harmful, and second, that they can facilitate weight loss. The reverse is true. Let's look at both of these issues.

First, a high-protein intake can be harmful. It often causes people to underconsume other essential nutrients, thus putting them at risk for other health problems.

Second, protein has no special power to promote weight loss. A "diet" only leads to loss of body fat *if* one eats fewer calories than needed to maintain body weight. Often diets high in a few foods tend to become boring, causing the dieter to eat less and less food. Weight loss, then, is due to consuming fewer calories, not to the protein. There can be some initial weight loss with these programs due to water loss. That weight loss, however, is often regained once the body has adjusted to the change in intake. Another claim for their use is that a high-protein, very-low-carbohydrate diet decreases one's insulin needs. For those who are overweight, the best way to decrease insulin needs and insulin resistance is to lose weight (10 to 20 pounds) and increase physical activity. For others of average or less weight, the above concerns should be considered—the negatives of omitting nutritious carbohydrate foods, and increasing fat intake.

These diets are highly discouraged. Only follow such a plan after checking with your doctor and making sure it is part of a supervised program that includes guidance by a registered dietitian, an exercise component, and frequent monitoring of laboratory values.

Vegetarian Food Plans

Vegetarians follow food plans that either limit or eliminate animal foods. Such a food plan can be successfully followed by someone with diabetes, and actually can be very positive healthwise. These food plans are typically low in saturated fat and high in whole grains, fruits, and vegetables. However, when one eliminates animal foods, certain nutrient requirements may be difficult to meet, including protein and vitamin B_{12}. Both of these can be met with carefully planning.

Vitamin B_{12} is in dairy and egg products, so consuming these protein sources typically can help you meet your B_{12} requirements. If you eliminate dairy and egg products, carefully read food labels and look for foods that have been fortified with B_{12}. (B_{12} is not naturally found in grain foods so it needs to be added.) Breakfast cereals, soy milk, and special vegetarian foods often have B_{12} added.

You can usually meet your protein needs by consuming a variety of nonanimal foods. The one concern is that of the 20 amino acids found in protein, there are nine that your body cannot make. These nine "essential" amino acids need to be consumed from the food you eat. All nine are found in animal foods—meat, poultry, fish, eggs, milk, yogurt, and cheese—which you may be eliminating. One plant food—soy—contains all nine essential amino acids. Other plant foods such as grains, dried beans and peas, nuts, and seeds do contain some of the nine, but not all nine essential amino acids in one food. By eating a variety of these foods through out the day, you can easily consume enough of the nine essential amino acids to meet your requirements.

PROTEIN AND KIDNEY DISEASE

Kidney disease is a concern when you have diabetes, and your primary care provider will monitor you closely for it. To prevent kidney disease or delay its onset, keep your blood glucose levels as close to normal as possible, control your blood pressure, and don't smoke.

The general nutrition guidelines, with an emphasis on whole grains, fruits, and vegetables, for diabetes care will help you achieve good blood glucose and good blood pressure control. In addition, many people with high blood pressure need to reduce their intake of sodium.

The first sign of kidney disease is "spilling" small amounts of protein into your urine (this is called microalbuminuria). Your kidneys filter your blood and allow waste to be excreted. When protein starts to be excreted in the urine, the kidneys are not properly filtering the urine.

Small amounts of protein can be detected by conducting a random test on a small amount of your urine, on a collection of urine over a limited period of time like 4 hours or overnight, or on a 24-hour collection. It is recommended that two or three tests be done over three to six months before diagnosing microalbuminuria. The laboratory doing your test will tell you the normal range for the type of test you have done. Often, if you have 30–300 mg albumin in a 24-hour collection, you are considered to have microalbuminuria.

When protein starts to spill into the urine, it is time to decrease dietary protein intake. The recommendation would then be to consume about 10% of calories from protein. To quickly know how much protein this is, look at the table on page 144. The range of protein for the different calorie levels is 15–20%; 10% would be half of the 20% amount. For an 1,800-calorie intake 10% would be half of 90 grams—45 grams.

You can also calculate your reduced protein needs by figuring 0.8 grams per kilogram of your body weight, or 0.4 grams of protein per pound of body weight. For a 150-pound person this would be 55 grams (based on 0.8 g/kg) to 60 grams (based on 0.4 g/pound) of protein a day.

CHAPTER 12

Learning about Fats

The first thing to know about fats is that you *do* need them. Fat is very important in helping your body work smoothly, and it adds a certain taste to foods. That said, you have most likely heard many times that you should eat less fat. That's because most Americans *do* eat too much fat. Excess fat contributes to two health problems connected to diabetes—weight gain and risk of heart disease. Several new health programs focus specifically on the importance of monitoring blood fat levels, as well as blood glucose levels in all persons with diabetes. The information in this chapter is very important to understand and use. This chapter will:

- Explain the role of fat in a diabetes food plan
- Identify sources of "good" and "bad" fat
- Provide recommendations for choosing foods that contain fat

WHAT YOU SHOULD KNOW ABOUT FAT

Fats help your body operate smoothly, and give you nutrients and essential fatty acids. Additionally, stored body fat protects your body's organs such as your liver, pancreas, and heart. However, you only need a limited amount of fat to meet your nutritional needs and protect your body. Once your fat and calorie needs are met, excess fat can contribute to health problems such as weight gain, hypertension, cardiovascular disease, and some cancers.

Fat is found in high amounts in shortening, butter, margarine, oils, bacon, whole milk, cheese, fatty meats, skin of poultry, and bakery items and many desserts.

Following are the most important points about fat intake and diabetes.

- *Do not eliminate all fat from your diet.* Some nutrients are only found in fat and cannot be made by the body. These are the essential fatty acids, including linoleic acid, linolenic acid, and arachidonic acid for infants.
- *Fat intake does count.* Many people with diabetes count their carbohydrate choices, but not their fat at meals and snacks. However, too much fat can cause weight gain, and too much saturated fat can raise blood cholesterol levels.
- *Decrease your intake of saturated fat.* Some fats will do damage in your body, while others seem to be protective or neutral fats. Saturated fats contribute to high cholesterol levels and should be consumed in small amounts. Monounsaturated fats are the fats to choose most often for your fat choices.
- *Enjoy more food when you follow a low-fat food plan.* When you replace high-fat foods with other food choices, you actually eat a larger quantity of food for the same number of calories.
- *Be aware that low-fat and reduced-calorie foods may contain extra carbohydrate.* When fat is reduced or removed from a food, special ingredients are added to replace the characteristics, such as a smooth texture, that fat typically provides. These ingredients often contain carbohydrate. Read the nutrition facts panel to learn how much extra carbohydrate to count in your food plan.
- *Know that a high-fat meal can affect your blood glucose level.* A high-fat meal is more slowly digested than a lower-fat meal. That means your blood glucose will rise later after a high-fat meal because the digestion of carbohydrates will be delayed. If your

blood glucose is typically down to your target range about two hours after you eat, it may be higher later after a high-fat meal. Make a note in your record book when you have more fat than usual and see if your blood glucose follows this pattern.

HOW MUCH FAT TO EAT

Two important considerations when choosing how much fat to eat are (1) the type of fat you use and (2) whether you are on a weight management program or not.

The type of fat you choose is important because some fats cause damage and others do not. If you choose the "good" monounsaturated fats, your fat intake can be higher. That's because it does not do the damage other fats do. However, if you are trying to lose weight or maintaining your weight on a weight-management program, you will want to limit the intake of all types of fat. A small amount of fat has a lot of calories. If you eat extra calories from fat you may need to severely limit the other food you eat. Fat intake can be 20–35% of total calories.

A typical fat intake is 30% of total calories. The following table shows how many calories and how many grams of fat this is for different calorie intakes.

Amount of Fat at Various Calorie Levels When Fat Is 30% of Total Calories

Daily Calorie Amounts	1,200	1,500	1,800	2,000	2,500
Calories from fat	360	450	540	600	750
Grams of fat	40	50	60	65	80

Fats are commonly divided into categories—saturated or unsaturated—based on their structure. Their structure either makes them solid or liquid at room temperature. As you can imagine, different kinds of fats act differently in your body, and some are better choices than others.

Unsaturated Fats

Unsaturated fats (primarily oils) are liquid at room temperature. There are two types of unsaturated fats—monounsaturated and polyunsaturated.

Monounsaturated Fats

Monounsaturated fatty acids are sometimes called MUFAs (moo-fahs). These fats are getting a lot of attention these days and are considered neutral fats healthwise. In fact, these are the fats that are being recommended to be used in cooking, baking, and spreads in place of other fats (when possible) for a heart-healthy food plan. Foods high in MUFAs are canola, olive, and nut-based oils; olives; nuts; avocados; seeds; and peanut butter.

Polyunsaturated Fats

Polyunsaturated fatty acids are nicknamed PUFAs (poof-fahs). They are liquid or soft at room temperature and are found in vegetables and fish. Foods high in polyunsaturated fats include plant oils— corn, cottonseed, safflower, soybean, and sunflower oil; nuts— almonds, peanuts, walnuts, and sesame oil; and liquid or soft margarine and mayonnaise. One type of PUFA is omega-3 fatty acid. It is found in fatty fishes like salmon and tuna, herring, and mackerel, and is believed to help in lowering triglycerides levels.

Trans-unsaturated Fats

Trans-unsaturated fats are sometimes called trans fats. You might think of them as fats in transition—ones that have moved from one place to another. What has happened is that their structure has changed: they were liquid and now they are firmer.

Trans-unsaturated fats are unsaturated fats (oils) that have had hydrogen added to make them solid at room temperature. The oils have been *hydrogenated*. Margarine is an example; when you read a margarine ingredient label, it will tell you what kind of oil was used to make the margarine.

It is difficult to know the amount of trans fat in a food, because, currently, it is not listed in the nutrition facts panel of a food label as are the other types of fat. If you want to decrease your intake of trans fats, limit your intake of foods that contain hydrogenated fats. They are listed in the ingredient list as "hydrogenated fats" or "partially hydrogenated oils" and are in many snack foods. Use these foods in small amounts, or choose foods that have the hydrogenated oil listed later in the ingredient list, or not at all. When choosing a margarine, choose a spread that is made with yogurt or stanols, or a less firm margarine, like those in a tub or a squeeze bottle.

Saturated Fats

Saturated fats, such as butter and animal fat, are hard at room temperature. Hard fats like meat fat and shortening are the fats that tend to build bumps and clumps in your blood vessels, making it difficult for your blood to flow smoothly. Saturated fat is the type of fat that does the most damage to your body, especially to your heart and blood vessels. It has also been connected to some forms of cancer. You may like the taste of these fats, but once you realize how harmful they are to you, you will consider more strongly the need to avoid them or consume them in small amounts (see the following table).

Eat Fewer Foods That Contain Trans and Saturated Fat

Trans Fat	Saturated Fat
Hydrogenated fats and oils often in:	Whole milk:
• Bakery items	• Butter
• Cakes	• Cream
• Candy	• Cheese
• Chips	• Cream cheese
• Cookies	• Sour cream
• Crackers	Meat fat:
• Fast food	• Lard
• Margarine, stick	• Bacon fat
• Muffins	• Sausage
• Peanut butter, made with hydrogenated oil	• Fat from beef, chicken, ham, lamb, pork, and turkey
• Vegetable shortening	Some plant oils:
	• Coconut and coconut oil
	• Palm oil

Fat Replacers

It is not always simple to decrease or replace fat in foods. Fat contributes a variety of pleasing characteristics to a food, including taste, flaky texture, creamy mouth feel, smell, moistness, and tenderness. In an effort to reduce the amount of fat in various foods, food scientists have developed special low-fat ingredients. These ingredients are not typically available for home use, but are used by food manufacturers.

Names of fat replacers that you will see on an ingredient list include caprenin, carrageenan, cellulose gel, corn syrup solids, guar gum, hydrogenated starch hydrolysates (HSH), hydrolyzed corn starch, micropaticulated egg white and milk protein, modified food starch, pectin, polydextrose, olestra, and xanthan gum.

Fat replacers can be made from carbohydrate, protein, or fat. Most fat replacers are made from carbohydrates. It may seem confusing to have a fat replacer made from fat, but the kind of fat that is used is not fully digestable. That is how it reduces calories.

When a carbohydrate fat replacer is used, the calories and fat content are decreased, but the total amount of carbohydrate is increased. This may or may not be a big increase, and may or may not be of concern to you. The nutrition facts panel will tell you how much carbohydrate is in a food.

Usually the lower-fat version of a food item will be the healthier choice, but you will need to consider the additional carbohydrate in your total carbohydrate at a meal or snack. Chapters 6, 11, and 14 will help you monitor your carbohydrate intake.

BLOOD TESTS ON YOUR FAT LEVELS

Your doctor will measure your blood for levels of different kinds of lipids, or fat-like substances. Depending on the results, you may or may not need to adjust the type of fat you eat. The following table gives the recommended goals for these measurements and the following text describes each measurement in detail.

Recommended Levels for Blood Lipid Tests

Blood Test	Recommended Level
LDL cholesterol ("bad cholesterol")	Less than 100 mg/dl
HDL cholesterol ("good cholesterol")	Greater than 45 mg/dl for men Greater than 55 mg/dl for women
Total cholesterol	Less than 200 mg/dl
Triglycerides	Less than 150 mg/dl

Source: American Diabetes Association: "2002 Nutrition Recommendations for Diabetes Care," *Diabetes Care* 25, 2002 (S1).

Measuring LDL and HDL cholesterol levels is important for determining your risk of heart disease. The fat you consume combines with protein as it travels though your blood and to your cells. This traveling package is called lipo (fat) protein. There are different types of lipoprotein—some contain large amounts of cholesterol and some contain smaller amounts of cholesterol.

- Low-Density Lipoprotein (LDL) cholesterol carries cholesterol from the liver to other parts of your body. Some of its cholesterol can be left in your arteries, blocking your blood flow. It is often referred to as the "bad" cholesterol because it increases your risk of heart disease. Eating high amounts of saturated fat can raise your LDL cholesterol levels. Remember, your goal is lower LDL.
- High-Density Lipoprotein (HDL) cholesterol carries cholesterol from different parts of your body to the liver so it can leave the body. It is often called the "good" cholesterol and can decrease your risk of heart disease. Remember, your goal is higher HDL.
- Total cholesterol is the total amount of cholesterol from a blood sample. It includes both LDL and HDL cholesterol.
- Triglycerides are the storage form of fat. When your blood glucose is high and you do not have the right insulin balance your triglyceride levels may be high. For some people, eating high amounts of carbohydrate can increase their triglycerides levels.

FAT AND BLOOD GLUCOSE LEVELS

The amount of fat you eat can affect your blood glucose in two ways. First, excess fat intake can increase your body weight. Extra weight makes it more difficult to control your blood glucose because you are more insulin resistant.

Second, a high-fat meal can delay the digestion of your food so your blood glucose rises later than usual. This is of interest for those who are monitoring their post-meal blood glucose level (measured 2 hours after you start eating). You may have heard of the pizza experiment. This was done to evaluate the blood glucose rise after a high-fat meal. It was shown that the rise in blood glucose was delayed when high-fat pizza was eaten. This may help explain some high post-meal blood glucose levels you may have had.

Those who take insulin before each meal should know if a high-fat meal is affecting their blood glucose. Keep good records, noting when you have double or triple your usual amount of fat so you can adjust your insulin dose accordingly. For example, if you take a rapid-acting insulin and if you know your blood glucose rise will be later than usual, you may take your insulin after your meal rather than before your meal. This may help prevent a low-blood-glucose episode. Discuss this with your diabetes care team.

FAT AND HEART HEALTH

As a person with diabetes, you are at higher risk of developing heart disease than many who do not have diabetes. You can take steps to decrease this risk and prevent heart disease. If you already have a form of heart disease, these steps are still important for you as they can help prevent or delay further complications.

The first and most critical food-related step is to decrease your intake of saturated fat. The National Cholesterol Education Program (NCEP) and American Diabetes Association recommend that all persons with diabetes consume less than 10% of their calories from saturated fat. If your LDL level is above 100 mg/dl, lower that amount to 7% of total calories. The following table shows you how many grams of saturated fat this would be for different calorie amounts.

Amounts of Saturated Fat (Grams) That Are 10% and 7% of Total Calories for Different Daily Calorie Amounts

Calorie Level	1,200	1,500	1,800	2,000	2,500
10% (grams per day)	13	17	20	22	28
7% (grams per day)	9	12	14	15	20

It may seem a bit tedious to count the grams of saturated fat you eat, but this is a process you should do occasionally. In your food diary, write the amount of saturated fat next to each food or beverage you consume. To determine the amount of saturated fat in various foods use food labels, reference books on fat grams, or a website that helps you analyze your intake. Or have your dietitian help you, and also discuss what changes might help improve your fat choices.

Though it is more important to decrease your saturated fat intake, the NCEP still recommends that you limit your cholesterol intake to 300 mg per day. If your LDL is above 100 mg/dl, limit your cholesterol intake to 200 mg per day and limit your egg yolk consumption to three or four times per week. The amount of cholesterol per food serving is listed in the nutrition facts panel of the food label so you can add up your cholesterol grams as you check out your saturated fat intake.

Also if your LDL level is above 100 mg/dl, the NCEP also recommends that you eat 10–25 grams of soluble fiber and 2 grams of plant sterols or stanols a day.

Soluble fiber helps remove cholesterol from your body. It acts like a sponge soaking up cholesterol and removing it from your body. Foods high in soluble fiber are oats, barley, dried beans and peas;

some vegetables such as carrots, broccoli, brussels sprouts, and turnip greens; and fruits such as apples, oranges, pears, and strawberries.

Plant sterols and stanols limit cholesterol absorption. They are found in some nuts and seeds, but are most easily consumed from special food products. Several margarine-like spreads and salad dressings contain sterols and stanols. Examples are the brands Benecol and Take Control.

In addition to specific food modifications to decrease your risk for heart disease, managing weight, increasing physical activity, stopping smoking, and controlling blood pressure will also help.

FAT AND WEIGHT LOSS

Fat is so calorically dense that a small quantity can greatly increase your caloric intake. The following table compares two meals, illustrating that with a few changes you can easily decrease the number of calories you consume.

Calorie Comparison of a High-Fat Meal and a Low-Fat Meal

High-Fat Meal	Calories	Low-Fat Meal	Calories
1 cup whole milk	150	1 cup skim milk	90
1 extra crispy fried chicken breast	470	1 grilled skinless chicken breast	100
Lettuce salad	0	Lettuce salad	0
Caesar salad dressing, 2 Tbsp	150	Lite Caesar salad dressing, 2 Tbsp	60
1 cup mashed potatoes	150	1 cup mashed potatoes	150
Sour cream, 2 Tbsp	60	Fat-free sour cream, 2 Tbsp	35
Peach pie, ⅙	365	Peaches, ½ cup	60
Total calories	1,345	Total calories	495

FAT AND KETONE LEVELS

Has your doctor ever asked you to check your urine for ketones? When your body is not using blood glucose for energy and is instead using stored fat, one of the byproducts is ketones. Ketones can show up in both your blood and urine. Some people check their blood for ketones, but most check their urine with a special strip that is dipped in the urine.

Ketones are typically not a good sign. There are two primary reasons why your ketones might be high and you are using fat for energy: if you are not eating enough (starvation ketosis), or you do not have enough insulin and glucose cannot get into your cells to be used for energy (diabetic ketoacidosis).

Occasionally a small amount of ketones in the urine due to a sensible weight-loss program is acceptable. To determine which form of ketosis you have, check your blood glucose when you check your ketones. If your blood glucose is high (250 mg/dl or greater) and your ketones are moderate to large, contact your doctor immediately as you probably have diabetic ketoacidosis (DKA) and need more insulin. If you have type 1 diabetes, in severe cases you may have nausea and vomiting and need to go to an emergency room.

CHAPTER 13

Examining Vitamins, Minerals, and Other Dietary Supplements

D ietary supplements are available in many forms including tablets, capsules, powders, gel tabs, extracts, and liquids. They include vitamins, minerals, other nutrients, and herbal preparations as well as ingredients and extracts of animal and plant origin. The most common supplement is the multivitamin/mineral tablet or capsule.

This chapter will:

• Describe the role of key vitamins and minerals in diabetes
• Provide guidelines for using supplements

VITAMINS, MINERALS, AND DIABETES

Many vitamins and minerals have a role in blood glucose control (see the following table). It is important that your body has enough of these vitamins and minerals so it can work as efficiently as possible. You may wonder if you need to take a supplement of any special vitamin or mineral to help improve your blood glucose control. Right now, the American Diabetes Association states there is little research indicating that taking supplements of individual nutrients or blends of nutrients actually improves blood glucose control. More research needs to be done before we can confidently make that type of general recommendation.

Vitamins, Minerals, and Diabetes

Nutrient	Effect on Carbohydrate/Sugar Metabolism or Insulin	Effect of Taking Nutrient as a Supplement
Chromium	Helps make the glucose tolerance factor, which helps insulin function.	Supplementation may improve blood glucose control if you have a chromium deficiency and impaired glucose tolerance. In a study done in China, at high levels [1,000 ug] chromium picolinate improved A1C, blood glucose, insulin, and cholesterol levels in persons with type 2 diabetes.
Magnesium	Helps blood glucose cross-cell membranes and is part of enzymes involved in the body's use of sugar. Losing sugar in the urine may lead to excessive urinary losses of magnesium.	Those at risk of a deficiency should take supplements or magnesium chloride.
Zinc	Insulin is stored as inactive zinc crystals in the beta cells of the pancreas.	Moderate zinc deficiency may occur frequently in people with type 2 diabetes, but supplementation has not been shown to be beneficial or to have a positive effect on diabetes management.
Copper	Blood levels are higher in persons with retinopathy, high blood pressure, or large blood vessel disease. Without these complications, values are normal.	Supplementation is not recommended because of the possible effect of high insulin levels seen in persons with complications.

(continued)

Vitamins, Minerals, and Diabetes *(continued)*

Nutrient	Effect on Carbohydrate/Sugar Metabolism or Insulin	Effect of Taking Nutrient as a Supplement
Manganese	There is no evidence of diabetes affecting manganese.	Supplementation has not been shown to lower blood glucose levels.
Iron	Excess iron accumulates in the body if one has a disease called hemo-chromatosis. This disease is associated with impaired glucose tolerance.	Avoid iron supplements unless you are a woman of childbearing age or have been told you have or are at risk for iron deficiency anemia by your doctor.
Vitamin A	There is no correlation between vitamin A and A1C levels, although vitamin A plays a role in regulation of insulin secretion.	In rat studies, supplementation did not alter blood or urine sugar levels.
Niacin (nicotinic acid)	As a drug, niacin lowers cholesterol, VLDL, and triglyeride levels and raises HDL levels.	In drug form may lead to worsening of blood glucose control.
Nicotinamide	Research is being done to determine if large doses of nicotinamide can prevent or delay type 1 diabetes.	Should be avoided by persons with liver disease, it can cause skin changes, stomach problems, and it interacts negatively with some other medicines. Not currently recommended.
Thiamin	Daily requirements depend on amount of carbohydrate consumed.	Supplementation has no demonstrated effect on diabetes management.
Pyridoxine, Vitamin B_6	Deficiency in animals and humans has been associated with impaired glucose tolerance and impaired secretion of insulin and glucagons. Poor diabetes control may decrease levels of vitamin B_6.	Supplementation has no demonstrated benefits on blood glucose. Has been used to treat diabetic neuropathy, but better medications are available. Mega-doses are asso-ciated with toxic effects including neuropathy.

Nutrient	Effect on Carbohydrate/Sugar Metabolism or Insulin	Effect of Taking Nutrient as a Supplement
Vitamin C	Has a chemical structure similar to glucose. Chronic high-blood-glucose levels deplete body stores. Consuming large doses may interfere with blood glucose checks.	Supplementation (500 mg/day) did not affect blood glucose levels; avoid high intake levels.
Vitamin D	Persons with diabetes found to have reduced bone mass and mineral content. Low levels of vitamin D can cause this.	Supplementation has no demonstrated effect on diabetes control.
Vitamin E, Tocopherols	Vitamin E is a strong antioxidant and people with diabetes may have higher requirements for antioxidants.	Usefulness is unproven; there is concern about long-term toxicity of antioxidant supplements.
Vanadium Vanadate	In animal studies, large doses improved blood glucose.	Vanadium should be considered a prescription drug rather than a supplement.

Source: Adapted from Franz, M: "Micronutrients and diabetes." In *American Diabetes Association Guide to Medical Nutrition Therapy for Diabetes*, MJ Franz, JP Bantle, Eds. American Diabetes Association, Alexandria, Virginia, 1999.

However, there are times when you might want to consider taking a multivitamin plus mineral supplement, or take supplements of particular vitamins or minerals. Three such times follow:

- When your diabetes is not in good control. Research shows that this may cause some nutrient deficiencies. A multivitamin plus mineral supplement is recommended.
- When you are restricting calorie or carbohydrate intake. Because you may be eating less food or a smaller variety of foods, it may be difficult to consume the mix of foods you need to meet your nutrient needs. For some, taking a multivitamin

plus mineral supplement is like an insurance policy; you are adding a little extra protection.

- When you have difficulty consuming certain foods such as those high in calcium or iron and need a supplement to meet your daily requirements. However, do not consume more than 100% of the daily value (listed as %DV on the supplement label) unless you have discussed this with your dietitian and doctor.

If you choose to take a supplement, know that the supplement cannot replace a healthy diet. By choosing a variety of foods with an emphasis on whole grains, fruits and vegetables, and low-fat foods you can often meet your nutrient needs without supplements. It is the combination of foods you eat and the combination of nutrients the food provides that help your body work smoothly and efficiently.

GUIDELINES FOR USING SUPPLEMENTS

Use all supplements carefully, especially those that we know less about, including herbal and other botanical supplements. Several guidelines for selecting or using a supplement include:

- Discuss its use with your dietitian and doctor as the supplement may affect other conditions or medications you are taking.
- Keep records of your supplement use (see the following chart).
- Add one supplement at a time so you know what its effect is.
- Never substitute a supplement for a prescription drug without first checking with your doctor.

The International Diabetes Center's *A Guide to Herbs and Supplements in Diabetes* explores these supplements in detail including remedies for diabetes and heart health and buying tips. Order the booklet online at www.internationaldiabetes.com or call 1-888-637-2675.

THE MINERAL SODIUM

Since many people with diabetes have high blood pressure, it is important to know more about the mineral sodium. A recent study clearly shows that specific food choices can lower blood pressure.

My Nutritional Supplements—Vitamins, Minerals, Herbal, and/or Others		
Name of product/ company/ phone #		
List of ingredients		
Any precautions about its use?		
When did you start taking?		
When and how do you take it?		
Why are you taking it?		
Any changes since taking it? Side effects? Effects on blood glucose?		

The diet that produced the greatest reduction in blood pressure is called the DASH diet. DASH stands for the name of the study—Dietary Approaches to Stop Hypertension.

Hypertension is often defined as a blood pressure greater than or equal to 140/90 mmHg. The blood pressure goal for adults who have diabetes, however, is lower—less than 130/80 mmHg.

The DASH diet was compared to a typical American diet and was found to decrease blood pressure both in people who already had high blood pressure and in those who did not currently have it. Therefore, the DASH diet can help prevent high blood pressure and is worth adopting even if you have normal blood pressure now.

The DASH diet is rich in fruits, vegetables, and low-fat dairy foods and reduces total and saturated fat. It also is low in red meat, sweets, and sugar-containing drinks. The food choices are high in potassium, calcium, magnesium, fiber, and protein. This food plan matches the nutritional recommendations of a diabetes food plan.

The sodium intake for the first study of the DASH diet was 3 grams a day (or 3,000 milligrams). According to the American Dietetic Association, this compares to the average sodium intake of 4–6 grams per day (or 4,000–6,000 milligrams).

The researchers did a follow-up study to determine if lowering the sodium intake could reduce blood pressure better. It did. Reducing sodium intake made the DASH diet even more effective at reducing blood pressure.

Sodium is found in salt, so cutting back on sodium means cutting back on salty foods. Foods will taste different, but most people who follow a low-sodium food plan adapt quite well to less salty foods in about two weeks. Some general guidelines for reducing sodium intake are given in the following table.

Tips for Reducing Sodium Intake

Tip	Action
Read the food label.	Choose foods that are "sodium free" or "low sodium." Choose foods that have less than 240 mg of sodium per serving.
Choose fresh or frozen vegetables rather than canned.	If you have canned vegetables, rinse them—put them in a colander and run water over them for a minute. Cook them in fresh water.
Do not add salt when cooking foods like noodles, rice, and vegetables.	Omit all salt or decrease gradually.
Reduce the salt in most recipes by half.	Cut the salt in a recipe by half, then the next time you make the recipe try reducing the salt again by half.
Do not add salt to your food.	You can gradually use less salt at the table. Shake salt into your hand so you can see how much you are using. Gradually use less and less.
Instead of salt, use other flavorings and spices, such as lemon juice, salt substitute, and herbs.	Many cookbooks list suggestions for using flavorings and spices.

PART FIVE

Planning Your Meals

CHAPTER 14

Discovering Carbohydrate Counting

T his chapter helps you:

- Design your own carbohydrate counting food plan
- Adjust carbohydrate and insulin based on blood glucose levels

THE GOAL OF CARBOHYDRATE COUNTING

The goal of basic carbohydrate counting is to eat a similar amount of carbohydrate at each meal from one day to the next. This helps you control and manage your blood glucose more easily than if you ate random amounts of carbohydrate throughout the day.

With carbohydrate counting you will know how many "carbohydrate servings" or "carbohydrate grams" you are to have at each meal. This is the foundation to carbohydrate counting—your number of servings or grams. For example, if you eat three servings of carbohydrate for breakfast on Monday, then this is the amount you would eat for breakfast each day of the week. Consistency is the key.

COUNTING CARBOHYDRATE BY SERVINGS

Counting carbohydrate by servings is often how one starts a carbo-hydrate counting food plan. Servings help you become familiar with carbohydrate foods and their portion sizes.

To use this plan, you need to know how much food is equal to one serving. Consider this: if you didn't know how large a serving was and you were to choose four carbohydrates servings for a meal, you could eat a whole plate of potatoes, a loaf of bread, a jar of apple-sauce, and a gallon of milk. Obviously, this would be too many car-bohydrate servings for anyone! It is important to know the amount of food that equals one serving.

If you start counting carbohydrate by number of servings, you will eventually find that some foods you want to eat are not on the lists in appendix G. What should you do? Using the food label, you can easily figure out the portion size that equals one serving. Remember that about 15 grams of carbohydrate equals one serving.

Use the label information to figure out what serving size has 15 grams of carbohydrate. When you do this, you will find that it is not always easy to get one serving of a food to equal exactly 15 grams of carbohydrate. What if a serving has 11 grams or 20 grams of carbohydrate?

This illustration shows an example of a food label. This label tells you that 5 crackers give you 11 grams of carbohydrate. Would you count that as one serving? Look at the follow-ing table for guidelines to help you make this decision. According to this table any serving that contains between 11 and 20 grams of carbohy-drate counts as one serving.

Nutrition Facts
Serving Size: 5 crackers
Servings Per Container: About 30

Amount Per Serving

Calories 70

Total Fat 2g

Sodium 220mg

Total Carbohydrate 11g

Dietary Fiber 0g

Protein 1g

Simplified saltine crackers food label

Determining Carbohydrate Servings
from Grams of Carbohydrate

Grams of Carbohydrate	Count As
0–5	Free food (limit to 3–4 a day)
6–10	½ serving
11–20	1 serving
21–25	1½ servings
26-35	2 servings
36–40	2½ servings
41–50	3 servings
51–55	3½ servings
56–65	4 servings

Source: American Diabetes Association.

A special note about the range of carbohydrate in a serving: You may feel that is a bit unfair to count 11 grams of carbohydrate as one serving when you could eat more crackers and go up to 20 grams of carbohydrate, and still be eating one serving of carbohydrate. That is true. Each cracker has about 2 grams of carbohydrate, so you could eat 4 more crackers for a total of 9 crackers and still be eating one serving of carbohydrate.

Factors to consider when deciding whether to eat closer to 20 grams of carbohydrate for each of your servings include how hungry you are, and whether eating the larger portion will affect your blood glucose or weight.

Usually if you are counting carbohydrate servings you do not need to be concerned about the extra carbohydrate you consume as long as you are using the ranges in the previous table. If you need to be more precise with your carbohydrate intake, you can count carbohydrate by grams. In regard to weight, you will be eating a few more calories, but it may or may not affect your weight loss or weight maintenance. Your choices may balance out if you have some servings at the lower end of the carbohydrate range and some at the higher end. More importantly for weight management, you will need to monitor your fat and protein choices because they do contribute calories, even if they don't contain carbohydrate.

COUNTING CARBOHYDRATE BY GRAMS

Another way to guide your carbohydrate intake is to count carbohydrate grams. This is very similar to counting servings. For example, instead of choosing four servings of carbohydrate for lunch you would choose 60 grams of carbohydrate (4×15 grams = 60 grams). Try to stay within 5–7 grams of your target goals for grams at each meal. See the following table for guidelines. Some people find gram counting more convenient to use than counting servings. They use the number of grams in a serving of food from the food label and keep a running total until they meet their goal for that meal.

Carbohydrate Ranges per Serving

Carbohydrate Servings	Target Total Grams of Carbohydrate	Acceptable Range of Total Grams of Carbohydrate
½	6–7	6–7 grams
1	15	8–22 grams
2	30	23–37 grams
3	45	38–52 grams
4	60	53–60 grams
5	75	68–82 grams
6	90	83–95 grams

Source: American Diabetes Association.

A special note about the range of carbohydrate for a meal. The range of carbohydrate given in this table may seem wide to you. And it may be. How precise you need to be will depend on your blood glucose checks. Keep a record of what you eat, then check your blood glucose 2 hours after you eat. Do this for different amounts of carbohydrate and see if the range makes a difference to you.

Remember that there are a variety of factors that affect your blood glucose, including your activity, how far in advance of your meal you took your insulin, and the amount of fat in your meal. The carbohydrate ranges help emphasize that you do not need to be precisely exact with your food. And you cannot expect the precise, exact blood glucose response even if you eat the very same food on two different days.

KNOW YOUR SERVING SIZES

When counting carbohydrate servings or grams it is important to have the correct serving size. To know this you will need to know how to weigh and measure food. This may seem like something you may want to skip—but don't. Portion control is important.

Review and use the measuring tips in chapter 16 even if you are an experienced cook. When you measure, observe how much space foods take up on your dishes and in your bowls and glasses so you can eventually begin to eye-measure your portions. The eye-measuring guidelines given in the table on page 204 will be quite helpful.

It is easy to misjudge a serving size. When you are first diagnosed with type 2 diabetes, eating a fairly similar amount of carbohydrate is often sufficient to control your blood glucose levels. But later, as your diabetes has progressed and there is less insulin production and greater insulin resistance, being more exact with carbohydrate amounts becomes necessary.

Compare the two meals in the following table to see how easy it is to misjudge the amount of carbohydrate you eat.

There is a big difference in the carbohydrate content of the two meals, although looking at just the food one might think they are quite similar. It is easy to overeat unless you carefully monitor your serving sizes. Your blood glucose two hours after the meal will certainly be higher with the larger-carbohydrate meal.

Comparison of the Carbohydrate in Two Meals

Breakfast Goal: 3 servings of carbohydrate or 45 grams of carbohydrate

Meal 1	Servings	Grams	Meal 2	Servings	Grams
¾ cup dry cereal	1	15	1 bagel, regular	4	60
1 peach	1	15	1 9-in. banana	2	30
1 cup milk*	1	15	1 cup milk*	1	15
Totals	3	45	Totals	7	105

*You can count milk as 12 or 15 grams. It is usually rounded up to 15 grams.

As you become more comfortable with the carbohydrate content of various foods, you will soon be able to estimate the carbohydrate contents in mixed or combination foods such as homemade casseroles, soups, and desserts. There are many cookbooks that list the carbohydrate contents of recipes, and books with complied lists of convenience foods also list each food's carbohydrate content. Also, check the websites of fast-food and family-style restaurants for the carbohydrate content of their meals, or ask for this information at the restaurant. If a restaurant menu claims that a meal is low in calories or fat, the nutrient information needs to be available to the customer. Taking the time to find out carbohydrate contents will increase your comfort level when eating in a variety of situations.

DESIGNING YOUR FOOD PLAN

Your carbohydrate food plan will tell you how much carbohydrate to eat at each meal and snack. Knowing your usual eating pattern will help you design your carbohydrate counting food plan. You can use the food diary in chapter 3 and keep track of what you eat for 3–5 days, just to get started. Then, look over your diary and circle the foods that contain carbohydrate. You can use the quick guide to counting carbohydrates in the following table to help remind you what foods are high in carbohydrate.

Quick Guide to Carbohydrate Servings

Carbohydrate Food Type	One Serving (15 grams of carbohydrate)
Bread, cereals, grains, pasta, and rice	1 slice bread ½ small bagel ½ small hamburger or hot dog bun ½ cup cooked cereal ¾ cup unsweetened dry cereal 3 graham cracker squares 1 small biscuit, roll, or muffin 1 6-in. tortilla ⅓ cup pasta or rice

Carbohydrate Food Type	One Serving (15 grams of carbohydrate)
Starchy vegetables	½ cup potatoes, corn, or dried beans or peas
Fruit	½ cup fruit or fruit juice 1 small apple or orange
Milk	1 cup
Mixed dishes	½ cup casserole (macaroni and cheese, lasagna, tuna noodle) 1 cup soup (all types, unless just broth)
Sweets	½ cup regular Jell-O ½ cup regular soda 2 small cookies ½ cup ice cream

Summarize your carbohydrate intake in the spaces below based on your usual eating pattern. You can use either servings of carbohydrate or grams of carbohydrate. If your amounts vary, write a range of carbohydrates, such as 1–2 servings, or 15–30 grams. The following sections will help you understand more about servings and grams.

	Time of Meal or Snack	Amount of Carbohydrate
Meal 1	_____	_____
Meal 2	_____	_____
Meal 3	_____	_____
Snack(s)	_____	_____
Total	_____	_____

If you haven't yet kept a food diary, look at the table on page 120 in the carbohydrate chapter. It lists the servings of carbohydrate one would generally consume at different caloric intakes. Then, use the example in the table on page 121 to help you distribute your carbohydrate throughout the day.

If this is more complicated than you want to do on your own, a dietitian can easily talk to you about what foods you like to eat and develop a carbohydrate food plan for you to get you started. Then, use the plan for a week or so and let your dietitian know what works and doesn't work for you, and what questions you have about how to use it. Don't worry if it takes a few sessions to get comfortable with your plan; there is a lot to know and your dietitian can help make it easier.

A carbohydrate counting food plan might look like this:

Breakfast   2 to 3 carbohydrate servings
Lunch   3 to 4 carbohydrate servings
Dinner   3 to 4 carbohydrate servings
or   2 to 3 carbohydrate servings at each meal, and 1 to 2 carbo-
      hydrate snacks each day
or   30 grams of carbohydrate at breakfast
      45 grams of carbohydrate at lunch and dinner

WHAT ELSE TO EAT

You will want to eat more than carbohydrate foods at a meal. You need to include foods containing protein and fat in order to meet your nutritional needs. Chapters 11 and 12 on protein and fat will give you specifics, but you can basically plan for 0–1 *ounces* of protein food at breakfast, 2-4 ounces at lunch, and 2–4 ounces at dinner, and a total of 3–5 servings (often teaspoons) of fat a day. With a carbohydrate counting food plan you do not need to keep track of these foods, yet they may contain other nutrients you need to track later, such as calories, sodium, and saturated fat.

For now, as you are getting started with a carbohydrate counting food plan, just count your servings or grams of carbohydrate. The rest of your food choices will fall into place and you can review them at a later date to see if they are the right amounts for you. Tracking too many nutrients at one time may be confusing or overwhelming, so start with what is manageable for you right now, then build on that.

PATTERN MANAGEMENT

As you become more comfortable counting carbohydrate and checking your blood glucose, you will be able to observe the impact of what you eat on your blood glucose levels. Look at your diabetes records for patterns—when are your blood glucose checks in your target range? When are they high? When are they low?

You may notice the unexpected. For example, your blood glucose level two hours after breakfast on Monday may be within your target range but not after breakfast on Tuesday or Wednesday. There are a variety of reasons this could occur. Some that are food related include misjudging the carbohydrate content of foods or measuring incorrectly. Chapter 6 provides more insight into looking for and understanding patterns in your blood glucose records.

When your balance of carbohydrate and insulin is right (either the insulin you make or insulin you take), your blood glucose levels are more likely to be in the range you want. If they are not, you may need to redistribute your food, adjust your activity, or begin taking a diabetes medication or adjust the one you are taking. The following section reviews how you can adjust the amount of insulin you take to match how much carbohydrate you plan to eat. Let your dietitian help you review your blood glucose records and help you assess your patterns.

USING INSULIN-TO-CARBOHYDRATE RATIOS

This section elaborates on how to make insulin adjustments when you want to eat more or less food than usual, and also explains what you can do if your blood glucose is higher or lower than usual before a meal. Who might want to do this? Anyone who takes before-meal injections of a rapid- or short-acting insulin or anyone who is on an insulin pump may wish to do so. This is most likely a person with type 1 diabetes, but someone with type 2 diabetes may want to do it as well.

In order to make insulin adjustments based on what you eat and what your blood glucose is before a meal, you will need to gather some baseline information about how your body responds to food. Keep detailed records of what you eat, your blood glucose checks (before meals and two hours after you start eating), your activity, and other factors that may affect your blood glucose level. It helps if you follow a food plan with very little variation in the amount of carbohydrate, protein, and fat. Also, keep your activity similar from day to day. Do this for a week. Then, along with your diabetes team, review your diabetes records to observe your patterns.

Review your records for patterns such as:

- How your premeal blood glucose compares to your after-meal blood glucose. Check your blood glucose two hours after you start eating your meal.
- The amount of rapid- or short-acting insulin you take before each meal for each serving of carbohydrate or for every 15 grams of carbohydrate. Look at this for all your breakfast meals, then lunches, then dinners. Is there a pattern?

This type of information will help you establish guidelines for how to adjust your insulin when you eat more or less food. You can also learn how to adjust your insulin if your blood glucose is higher or lower than expected before a meal.

Adjusting Insulin for How Much You Plan to Eat

Learning how to adjust your insulin for the amount of food you plan to eat gives you a great deal of flexibility. It will take time to learn this, but most people who do say it is well worth the effort. Let's look at some examples.

Sam

Before lunch Sam takes three units of a rapid-acting insulin and eats three servings (45 grams) of carbohydrate. At two hours after he eats, his blood glucose is within his goal of less than 160 mg/dl. Sam figures that for every serving of carbohydrate (15 grams) he eats at lunch he needs one unit of insulin. Some days he likes to eat an extra serving of carbohydrate, so on those days he takes four units of insulin. By looking ahead Sam knew that the extra serving carbohydrate would raise his blood glucose, so he took an extra unit of insulin. Doing so helps him meet his blood glucose goals.

Jackie

Jackie has been trying to lose weight but finds when she eats less and takes her usual amount of rapid-acting insulin she has a low-blood-glucose episode. She then needs to eat in order to treat her low blood glucose. This means she is not losing weight. By looking ahead, Jackie began to plan for the lower rise in blood glucose that resulted when she ate less food. She took less insulin. She typically ate 3 servings (45 grams) of carbohydrate for lunch and wanted to now eat just one or two servings for lunch several days a week. On most days she took three units of insulin, but now is able to adjust this when she eats less: she takes one unit of insulin for every serving of carbohydrate she plans to eat.

These examples are based on how much insulin is needed to lower the blood glucose rise from a certain amount of carbohydrate. The rise in blood glucose is called "glucose excursion." You can adjust your insulin based on the expected glucose excursion. To do this, you first decide how much carbohydrate you are going to eat, then take enough insulin so that your blood glucose two hours after your meal will be within your target range.

In the above examples, Sam and Jackie both planned to take one unit of rapid-acting insulin for every serving of carbohydrate (15 grams) they ate at lunch. This is a common ratio, 1:15, and can be a starting point for you. Insulin-to-carbohydrate ratios may be different at different times of the day. You may need a unit of insulin for every 10 grams of carbohydrate in the morning, and at dinner you may need a unit for every 20 grams of carbohydrate. Review your diabetes records with your dietitian to see what patterns you observe.

Following are two guidelines that many health professionals use when someone begins to adjust insulin before meals, if diabetes records are not available or do not present a clear pattern.

1. Start by using one unit of insulin for every serving of carbohydrate (15 grams) you eat, or
2. Follow the Rule of 500

In the Rule of 500, you add up *all* the insulin units you take in one day and divide that total into 500. The answer you will get is the number of grams of carbohydrate to eat for each unit of insulin. For example, let's say you take 15 units of an intermediate-acting insulin, and your rapid-acting dosage is 4 units before breakfast, 5 before lunch, and 7 before supper.

- Add 15 + 4 + 5 + 7 and you get 31.
- Divide 500 by 31 and you get 16.

The Rule of 500 ends up with a similar starting point as the first guideline. The result of 16 is very close to 15, so you would use one unit of insulin for every 16 grams of carbohydrate you eat. These guidelines are just to get you started and soon you will learn if they are right for you by reviewing your blood glucose patterns.

Adjusting Your Insulin for High or Low Before-Meal Blood Glucose

You will most likely encounter situations where your blood glucose before a meal is a bit higher or lower than usual. You can adjust your insulin to correct for this. If your blood glucose is higher and you are eating your usual amount of food you will need to take a little extra insulin. Of course, it follows that if your blood glucose is lower than usual, you will need to take less insulin.

You will need guidelines for adjusting your insulin in these situations. Two of these will be presented here. They have been developed by health professionals as helpful guides and though they have not been widely researched, they are becoming widely used. You should be sure to discuss them and your calculations with your diabetes care team before making any changes in your insulin.

1,500 and 1,800 Guides

The first method is similar to the 500 method for determining your insulin-to-carbohydrate ratio (see page 180). This time you will use either 1,500 or 1,800, dividing one of these numbers by the total amount of insulin you take in one day. Some health professionals recommend 1,500 if you take short-acting insulin before your meals, and 1,800 if you take rapid-acting insulin before meals.

Let's say you take short-acting insulin, and your total insulin units for a day are 45; divide 1,500 by 45, which is 33 (round up to 35). The number 35 is used to correct for the high or low blood glucose. It means, on average, that for every 35 mg/dl your blood glucose is higher than your usual level, you will need to take one extra unit of insulin.

This may seem complicated at first, but it does get easier. You will need to know your correction factor (1,500 or 1,800 divided by total insulin dose), your blood glucose goal before your meals (values between 100 and 150 mg/dl are often used), and your before-meal blood glucose. This is the formula to use: subtract 150 from your current blood glucose level and then divide that value by your correction factor. The following is an example.

Let's say your blood glucose is 70 mg/dl over your before-meal blood glucose goal of 150 mg/dl. The correction factor in this example says that for every 35 mg/dl over 150 mg/dl you would need to take one extra unit of short-acting insulin. Divide 70 by 35 and you get 2; you need two additional units of insulin.

If you do not want to do the math every time your blood glucose is high or low, you can make an insulin adjustment table based on your correction factor. The table on the following page gives an example using the correction factor of 35 with short-acting insulin.

Insulin Adjustment When Using Short-Acting Insulin and Correction Factor of 35*

When Your Blood Glucose Is:	Your Correction Factor Is:	Take This Amount of Short-Acting Insulin:
70–150 mg/dl	—	5 units
151–185 mg/dl	+1 units	6 units
186–220 mg/dl	+2 units	7 units
221–255 mg/dl	+3 units	8 units
256–290 mg/dl	+4 units	9 units
291–325 mg/dl	+5 units	10 units

*This is only an example. You will need your own adjustment guide.

Following is an example of how to use insulin and carbohydrate information to help you reach your blood glucose goals.

Heidi

Heidi usually eats 45 grams of carbohydrate for breakfast. She takes one extra unit of rapid-acting insulin for every additional 15 grams of carbohydrate she eats. Her breakfast insulin-to-carbohydrate ratio is 1:15 and her correction factor is 33. Her fasting blood glucose goal is 70–140 mg/dl.

What should Heidi do if her fasting blood glucose is 172 and she plans to eat her regular breakfast? Heidi needs to use her correction factor and take extra rapid-acting insulin because her fasting blood glucose is 32 mg/dl above her target range. She takes one extra unit of rapid-acting insulin and eats her usual breakfast.

What should Heidi do if her fasting blood glucose is 172 and she wants to eat 60 grams of carbohydrate for breakfast? Heidi needs to use her correction factor to correct for the high fasting blood glucose, and add supplemental insulin for the extra food. She would take one extra unit of insulin for correction and one extra unit for the additional food. This is two extra units.

CHAPTER 15

Using the Exchange System

T he exchange system for meal planning helps persons with diabetes select food in appropriate quantities. It helps one *achieve a consistent intake of carbohydrate, protein, and fat from day to day.* Until carbohydrate counting became popular in the 1990s, the exchange system was the primary method of diabetes meal planning. It is still very useful and can even be used to teach carbohydrate counting.

This chapter will:

- Explain the exchange system
- Describe how an exchange food plan is developed
- Provide suggestions on how to use the exchange system for carbohydrate counting

UNDERSTANDING THE EXCHANGE SYSTEM

The exchange system is based on six food groups or "lists": starch/bread, meat and meat substitutes, vegetables, fruit, milk, and fat. Each food in a list is similar to other foods in that list. For example, all foods in the fruit list are fruits.

People using the exchange system consume foods from each list each day. But how much food? A food plan is designed to guide each individual so they can achieve the goal of having a consistent intake from day to day.

An exchange list food plan may look like this for breakfast:

Food List	Number of Servings at Breakfast
Starch	2
Fruit	1
Milk	1
Nonstarchy vegetables	0
Meat and substitutes	0–1
Fat	0–1

Looking at this plan you can imagine eating two slices of bread, a piece of fruit, a glass of milk, and a little margarine on your bread or toast. That would be correct, but you may wonder how this would work if you wanted cereal or pancakes. The following will describe each food list, and explain how you can vary what you eat and still be following your food plan.

THE EXCHANGE LISTS

Each food in an exchange list is similar in how much carbohydrate, protein, and fat it contains. For example, all fruits in the fruit list have a lot of carbohydrate and no protein or fat. Chicken, which is on the meat list, has *no* carbohydrate, a lot of protein, and some fat. This is the same composition as other foods on the meat and meat substitutes list. Foods in the fat list have a different composition; they contain no carbohydrate and no protein, just fat. Any food that contains mostly fat is listed in the fat list and includes such foods as butter, margarine, nuts, and mayonnaise.

Once foods have been categorized into a food list, they are given a serving size. Each serving has a similar amount of carbohydrate, protein, and fat. When carbohydrate, protein, and fat are the same, the calories will also be the same. In fact, because of this, even people without diabetes sometimes use the exchange lists for weight management. The following table lists the amount of carbohydrate, protein, fat, and calories in one serving from each food list.

Exchange List Food Groups

List	Carbohydrate per Serving (grams)	Protein per Serving (grams)	Fat per Serving (grams)	Calories per Serving
Carbohydrate Lists				
Starch	15	3	0–1	80
Fruit	15	0	0	60
Milk				
Skim or 1%	12	8	0–3	90
Reduced fat or 2%	12	8	5	120
Whole	12	8	8	150
Sweets, desserts, and other carbohydrates	15–30	2–4	5–10	80–205
Nonstarchy Vegetables	5	2	0	25
Meat and Substitutes				
Very lean meat and substitutes	0	7	0–1	35
Lean meat and substitutes	0	7	3	55
Medium-fat meat and substitutes	0	7	5	75
High-fat meat and substitutes	0	7	8	100
Fats				
Monounsaturated	0	0	5	45
Polyunsaturated	0	0	5	45
Saturated	0	0	5	45
Free Foods	less than 5 grams	0	0	less than 20

Source: Exchange Lists for Meal Planning. American Diabetes Association and American Dietetic Association, Chicago, Illinois, 2003; used with permission.

By looking at the table you can see the differences in the different food lists. You can see that fruit has a lot of carbohydrate and no protein or fat. Each serving of fruit in the fruit list provides 15 grams of carbohydrate. That is the convenience of the exchange system— the calculations are already done for you. For example, when looking at the fruit list for apples, pears, and watermelon, you will see the following servings; each contains 15 grams of carbohydrate and 60 calories.

Fruit	One Serving
Apple	1 small
Pears	½ large
Pears	½ cup, canned
Watermelon	1¼ cups, cubes
Apple Juice	½ cup
Grape Juice	⅓ cup

Most of the changes in the exchange lists over the years relate to fat. When the exchange lists were first designed there was not as much interest in fat content, and not as many reduced-fat food choices. There are now more categories in the milk and meat groups, and foods in the fat list are divided into monounsaturated fat, polyunsaturated fat, and saturated fat lists. This additional information helps those who are following a low-fat food plan or limiting certain types of fat.

The exchange lists in appendix G are from the American Diabetes Association and the American Dietetic Association. These two organizations also publish a booklet titled *Healthy Food Choices,* described in chapter 4. Its exchange lists are shorter and not quite as specific as the longer exchange lists. For example, in *Healthy Food Choices* all fruit juice servings are a half of a cup, yet from the above example you know that in the longer, more specific exchange lists, a serving of grape juice is one-third of a cup. There is not a lot of difference between these two servings sizes, and for many people with diabetes a general half-cup serving is easier to remember. Yet, for those who need to be more precise with their carbohydrate and calorie intakes, it can be quite helpful to have the more specific information. The lists from *Healthy Food Choices* are very similar to the lists from the Food Guide Pyramid on page 45.

GETTING STARTED

To start an exchange list food plan you will either use a predetermined plan, or more appropriately, a plan designed especially for you taking into account how, when, and what you like to eat. Before you can use an exchange food plan, however, you need to know what foods are in the different lists and the serving sizes of different foods.

Review the foods in the different food lists either in the table on page 45 or appendix G. You may be surprised that some foods are on a different list than you expected. For example, many think of corn as a vegetable (which it is), yet it is on the starch list. This is because it has a lot of carbohydrate, making it more similar in composition to foods in the starch list than lettuce and green beans on the vegetable list. Many think of bacon as meat, yet it is primarily fat, just like other foods on the fat list. Reviewing the lists will help you become familiar with what foods are on each list.

Once you have reviewed the foods in each list, look at the serving sizes. Each measurement is based on how much of a food meets the nutrient composition of that food list (the values in the previous table).

To keep each list manageable, not all foods are included in the lists. Many reference books and cookbooks list the nutrient content of additional foods as well as their exchange values. Some food labels will also list exchange values. You can use the information on the nutrition facts panel of a food label to determine how a food fits into the exchange system. Here's an example.

In the illustration on the next page, the granola bar's composition is very close to one serving from the starch list. Look at the amount of total fat, total carbohydrate, and protein on the food label and compare it to the values in the previous table. You can count the granola bar as one carbohydrate serving.

As you use food labels more you will have more questions about how to "count" a food. Two other tables will help you. These tables give ranges for how to decide if a food is one or more servings of carbohydrate or fat. The carbohydrate table on page 171 is in the carbohydrate counting chapter, and the other table is here.

Nutrition Facts

Serving Size: 1 bar
Servings Per Container: 1

Amount Per Serving

Calories 90

Total Fat 2g

Sodium 105mg

Total Carbohydrate 17g

    Dietary Fiber 1g

Protein 1g

Simplified granola bar food label

Determining Fat Servings from Grams of Fat

Amounts of Fat	Corresponding Serving Size
0–2 g	Do not count
3 g	½ fat serving
4–7 g	1 fat serving
8 g	1½ fat servings
9–12 g	2 fat servings
13 g	2½ fat servings
14–17 g	3 fat servings
18 g	3½ fat servings
19–22 g	4 fat servings

Source: American Diabetes Association.

The granola bar has two grams of fat. You do not need to count this fat according to the table above. If the granola bar had three grams of fat, this table suggests that you count that amount as a half of a fat serving. In reality, there are very few people who count half servings of fat. Yet, this information is very valuable especially for those who are on a weight-management plan. Every little bit of extra fat you eat quickly adds to your daily caloric intake. You can either count the half servings, or put that amount of fat into the lower or higher serving amount. If the fat grams was 13, you could count that as either two or three fat servings. Since these changes do not affect blood glucose control, you can be flexible with your counts, and have a daily fat total rather than being very precise at each meal.

Several general guidelines can help you with foods that combine foods from the different food lists. One general guide, for example, is that 1 cup of a casserole, lasagna, or macaroni and cheese is equal to two carbohydrate servings and two medium-fat servings. Another guide is that one-fourth of a 10-inch, thin-crust cheese pizza is two carbohydrates, two medium-fat meats, and one fat. More guidelines for combination foods are in appendix G. Some people with diabetes may need to be more precise with their measurements, but for most people these general guidelines are sufficient in helping them meet their diabetes nutrition goals.

DESIGNING YOUR FOOD PLAN

Your exchange system food plan will tell you how much to eat from each food group at each meal and snack. Keeping a food diary, as outlined in chapter 3, will help you design a plan based on how you usually eat.

To highlight the variety of meals you can have from a basic food plan, let's look at a sample plan for lunch:

Exchange List	Number of Servings at Lunch
Starch	2 servings
Fruit	1 serving
Milk	1 serving
Nonstarchy vegetables	1–2 servings
Meat and meat substitutes	2–3 servings
Fat	0–1 serving

There are many different meals that can be made from this basic plan. With this plan you could have a sandwich, piece of fruit, and a glass of milk. Or you could have two tacos, juice, and yogurt. Or a cup of tomato soup, crackers, cheese, canned fruit, and milk. The flexibility of food choices is one of the reasons the exchange system has been successful for so many years.

Standard exchange food plans have been developed and are sometimes handed out as tear-off diet sheets or published in books and magazines. These can be difficult to follow because they are not individualized to your personal eating pattern and food preferences, nor your activity and diabetes needs. However, for some, these sheets have helped them start following a diabetes food plan. The menus in chapter 5 are considered standard food plans and can serve as a guide for starting a diabetes food plan or provide menu suggestions that you can adapt to your own food plan. If a standard plan is what you are following now, consider consulting a dietitian to help personalize it.

Carbohydrate Exchanges

To help you have more flexibility with your exchange food plan, look again at the table on page 185 and notice that four of the food lists have been combined under the heading "carbohydrates." Each food in this group has more carbohydrate than protein or fat. Thus, they are primarily carbohydrate foods. Three of the lists—starch, fruit, and milk—have similar amounts of carbohydrate in one serving, 12–15 grams. For that reason, choosing between groups is acceptable. If you have the above food plan for lunch and do not want to choose one serving from the milk list, using the broad carbohydrate group, you could choose a serving from either the starch or fruit group.

If you like this type of planning, your food plan would look like this:

Exchange List	Number of Servings at Lunch
Carbohydrates (starch/bread, fruit, milk)	4 servings
Vegetables	1–2 servings
Meat and substitutes	2–3 servings
Fat	0–1 serving

You may wonder what to do about the vegetable list. Each serving only has 5 grams of carbohydrate. In the exchange system, any food that has less than 5 grams of carbohydrate or 20 calories per serving is a free food. Generally, one to two servings of vegetables are counted as "free." This is partly because vegetables are relatively low in carbohydrate and calories, and also to encourage you to eat more vegetables. If you have two servings (providing 10 grams of carbohydrate), you can check your blood glucose and see if that amount causes an extra rise after your meal. If so, you can decrease your intake of your other carbohydrate foods to accommodate the two servings of vegetables.

Another thing you may wonder about is the value of the exchange system over the carbohydrate-counting food plan as explained in chapter 14. As you may have noticed, there is a great amount of overlap between the two. The main difference is that the exchange system gives guidance in choosing noncarbohydrate foods—meats and meat substitutes and fat. This information is valuable to know for everyone with diabetes, even if following general guidelines or a plate method of meal planning.

Free Exchanges

Everyone loves "free foods." Appendix G contains a list of free foods. These are foods that contain less than 20 calories per serving and do not need to be accounted for when you eat them. It is usually recommended that free foods be limited to three or four servings a day, and not eaten all at one time. You can use free foods and foods from the vegetable list to extend other foods you choose to eat. Some examples of extending are:

- Fruit in calorie-free gelatin
- Fruit juice mixed with club soda or fizzy water
- Large lettuce salad with chicken, cottage cheese, or tofu
- Clear broth soup with chunks of celery, tomato, and zucchini, and potato or rice

- Fat-free mayonnaise mixed with horseradish for a spicy sandwich spread

Becoming familiar with the food lists will help you put together creative, tasty meals and low-calorie meal extenders.

PART SIX

Tips for Choosing Foods

CHAPTER 16

Enjoying Meals Away from Home

Have you ever felt that you should eat all your meals at home so you can better control the food you eat? No one should feel so confined or limited because of diabetes. With the tips provided in this chapter you can feel more confident and in control when eating away from home.

This chapter discusses how to:

- Make adjustments if there are changes in your mealtimes
- Be in charge of the food you eat when eating away from home
- Use alcohol appropriately

CHANGES IN MEALTIMES

As part of your diabetes food plan, you will have designated times for when you plan to eat. But what do you do if your mealtime needs to be changed? Eating 30 minutes to 1 hour before or after your designated mealtime usually causes no problem with blood glucose control. However, eating a meal more than an hour earlier or later may affect your blood glucose control. This can happen more frequently when you eat a meal away from home than when you eat at home.

Your meals are typically spaced to allow your blood glucose to return to a target range before meals. If you eat early, your blood glucose may still be high from the previous meal. And if you eat late, your blood glucose might be too low before the meal. For some, this balance is more delicate than for others. You will need to learn how to make the adjustments that are best for you.

The following general guidelines will help you prepare for early or delayed meals. If a general guideline does not work for you, you will have to individualize your plans based on your blood glucose records. Your individual changes will depend on:

- How much carbohydrate you eat at each meal
- Whether you eat snacks or not
- What your activity schedule is
- What your target blood glucose goals are
- If you take a diabetes medications, what type of diabetes medicine you take, when you take it, and how much you take

Guidelines for Early Meals

Various situations may require you to eat a meal more than an hour earlier than your scheduled time. In general, follow these steps:

- Eat the meal early, but save one starch, fruit, or milk serving (15 grams of carbohydrate) to eat at your regular mealtime.
- If you usually take a diabetes medication before your regular mealtime, you would also usually take it before the early meal. This may affect your blood glucose levels later in the day. To be sure, review your medication plan with your diabetes care team ahead of time to determine how to adjust your diabetes medicine for early meals.

Guidelines for Delayed Meals

Delayed or late meals are common when eating at friends' houses or restaurants. Traveling or traffic jams may also delay meals. General guidelines for delayed meals include:

- At your regular mealtime, have one starch, fruit, or milk serving (15 grams of carbohydrate). Eat the rest of your meal later.
- If you usually have a snack at the later time, eat the snack at the regular mealtime and the meal at the snack time.
- If you take a diabetes medication, it is safest to take it before the later meal, but this may affect your blood glucose levels later. Again to be sure of the best change for you, review your medication plan with your diabetes care team ahead of time to determine how to adjust your diabetes medicine for delayed meals.

Insulin and Changed Meal Times

Changed meal times are the most challenging when you take insulin. The most important consideration is to prevent a low-blood-glucose episode with a changed mealtime, especially with a delayed meal. Knowing the action of your insulin will help you make any necessary food changes. Review the action of your insulin regimen in chapter 2 and note when it begins to work and when it is peaking, then discuss changing meal times with your dietitian or others on your diabetes care team.

Always have some food available in case of an unplanned delayed meal. Keep food handy at work, at school, in the car, and with you while you travel. See the following table for a list of travel snacks that are already packaged and ones that can easily remain fresh in plastic containers. One serving, or 15 grams of carbohydrate, may be all you need to eat before your delayed meal. However, if you are driving, be sure you eat enough so you do not have a low-blood-glucose episode. Instead of delaying your meal, you may want to make a meal out of these snacks. If you want, you can keep on hand canned tuna, low-fat jerky, and nuts and seeds including walnuts, peanuts, and sunflower or soy seeds to add to the portable snacks.

Easy Portable Snacks

Snack Type	Amount Equal to 15 Grams Carbohydrate
Beverages or sports drink	1 cup
Fruit or vegetable juice	½ to 1 can or box
Cereal	¾ to 1 cup
Cereal or granola bars	1
Cookies or crackers	
Ginger snaps	3
Oreo-style	2
Vanilla wafers	5
Animal crackers	7
Graham	3 squares
Goldfish	½ cup
Oyster	26
Soda or saltines	6
Crackers and cheese or peanut butter sandwiches	½ to 1 pack
Gummy bears	6
Raisins and other dried fruit	2 tablespoons
Canned fruit	½ cup or small container
Marshmallows	3 large
Pudding	1 small container
Rice cakes	5 mini cakes
Pretzel sticks	35
Pretzel rods	2½

Meal Times on Weekends versus Weekdays

You may want to eat at different times on the weekends than on weekdays. You can design two different schedules that easily let you move back and forth between these mealtimes. To begin, use the above guidelines for early and delayed meals.

If you take insulin and want to sleep late and delay breakfast more than 2 hours, discuss this with your diabetes care team. Depending on your insulin regimen, you may not be able to sleep late, or you need to set an alarm and take your intermediate-acting or long-acting insulin as well as 15 grams of carbohydrate, such as a half-cup of juice, near your usual mealtime. Checking your blood glucose to see if you are higher or lower than usual is suggested so you can adjust the amount of food you eat at this time. Then you can go back to sleep. When you get up, you can take your rapid- or short-acting insulin and eat the rest of your breakfast. Discuss options with your diabetes care team.

Swing Shifts and Night Shifts

Your meal times may change because of changes in your work hours or shifts, and this may require changes in your diabetes treatment plan. It is most important to take the time to develop a plan for swing shifts when you take a diabetes medication. The most efficient way to decide when to eat and take your diabetes medication is to start by drawing two horizontal lines across a piece of paper (see the illustration).

8 am	12	4	8	12	4	8 am

8 am	12	4	8	12	4	8 am

On one line, put a mark at the times you usually eat, and then do the same on the other line for the other days. If you have a third variation to your schedule, draw a third line and place marks when you eat and take your diabetes medication. You may be surprised at how close the mealtimes may match. If they do not, take this chart to your dietitian and doctor and discuss the time differences and possible medication adjustments.

If you take a diabetes medication, and the mealtimes on the different days are close, your medication may be taken as usual.

However, your activity may vary between the days, so either an adjustment in the amount of food you eat or the amount of medication you
take may be needed. Do some problem solving with your dietitian so
you will feel comfortable making any changes you need to make.

Traveling

Traveling to other states or other countries may be a routine part of
your work, or part of an exciting vacation. Having diabetes should not
limit your travel. The information in this book will help you deal with
many different situations—eating at restaurants, planning meals, stay-
ing active, preparing for sick days, and adjusting meal times.

The two main principles of a diabetes food plan remain important as you travel—have regular meal times and eat consistent
amounts of food. Traveling may pose challenges with both of these.
Your diabetes team can help you learn more about food choices at
your destination and help you make medication adjustments if you
are traveling through several time zones.

Carry your diabetes supplies with you whenever you travel. This
includes enough food for several snacks, bottled water, your blood
glucose meter and supplies, and your medicine. The supplies need to
be near you, not with checked luggage on an airplane or in the trunk
of a car. They need to be accessible and not placed where your supplies could get too hot or too cold.

The American Diabetes Association's *Diabetes Travel Guide* gives
additional travel guidelines including going on cruises and scuba
diving, and lists important phrases you may need in seven foreign
languages.

DIFFERENT EATING SITUATIONS

When eating away from home, it is still possible to be in charge of
the food you eat. At first glance, you may wonder how this can be. If
you are not cooking, how can you be in charge? Well, being in charge
means making informed decisions about what you eat. This means

that you will need to ask questions about the foods on the menu and make sure you have food available that fits your meal plan. The following guidelines can help you be comfortable in a variety of different eating situations.

Tips for Eating at a Friend's Home

When invited to a friend's house for a meal, let your friend know that you'd love to accept the invitation but, because you have diabetes, you have a couple of questions. Usually your host or hostess will be delighted to discuss the menu with you, and may ask you for suggestions. This is preferable for both you and your host than discovering right before the meal that it will be difficult for you to follow your food plan. Difficulties arise either because you don't know how a food has been prepared, you are unable to accurately estimate your portion size, or there is extra carbohydrate or fat in the food.

To help avoid surprises, ask the following questions a day or two before the meal:

- What time will the meal be served? Do not hesitate to explain what time range will be best for you, and use the above guidelines for early or delayed meals.
- What will be on the menu? If you are unclear as to what a food contains, ask how it is prepared so you can figure out how it can best fit your meal plan.
- May you bring an appetizer or dish to share? If this is possible, you will be able to prepare a food that either fits your food plan or contains little or no carbohydrate so you can freely munch on it.

Tips for Eating at Restaurants

Before going to an unfamiliar restaurant, feel free to call and ask for a description of some of the foods on their menu. You could pick up a menu at the restaurant, someone at the restaurant may be able to fax you a menu, or you may be able to review the menu on an internet site. Your goal is to know in advance what your choices are. Planning ahead usually makes the situation more comfortable and allows you to make the best choices for you. You will be more in control of the situation, which then puts you in control of your blood glucose.

General Restaurant Tips

Know your food plan and how different foods fit it.

- Call the restaurant in advance and ask how different menu items are prepared, or ask your server when you arrive.
- Become familiar with foods that will be served and look them up in an exchange booklet, or a carbohydrate/fat guidebook (also see appendix G).
- Ask if it is possible to order items that may not be on the menu, but that are used as ingredients in foods on the menu, such as fresh berries, cantaloupe, fresh spinach, red peppers, or celery.
- Carry a copy of your food plan with you as a reminder of your portion sizes.

Know how to avoid extra fat.

- Avoid foods that are fried, seasoned with fat, or have added gravies or creamy sauces.
- When possible, ask that oil, margarine, and butter be omitted or reduced in the preparation of your food.
- Ask for gravies, sauces, dressing, mayonnaise, butter, margarine, sour cream, and guacamole to be served on the side.
- Request low-calorie dressings and sour cream.
- Choose foods that are baked, broiled, boiled, steamed, or grilled.

Take control of how much you eat.

- Order a low-fat appetizer for your main meal rather than a meal entrée.
- Share an entrée or ask for half servings so you are not tempted to eat too much.

Restaurant Food Suggestions

Food Type	Suggestion
Appetizer	You may want to choose a low carbohydrate food so you can save your carbohydrate for your main meal or possibly dessert. Good choices are raw vegetables, such as carrots, celery, or radishes; fat-free, chicken, or beef broth; or vegetable soup. Ask if such items are available if you don't see them on the menu.
Salad	Choose vegetable salads with vinegar or lemon juice or a low-calorie dressing if available. Avoid croutons, as they are high in carbohydrate and fat.
Soup	Choose bouillon, broth, or consommé-based soups. Cream soups are high in fat. All soups are usually high in sodium.
Sandwiches	Chicken, turkey, low-fat cheese, and lean meat are good choices for fillings. Salad-type fillings made with mayonnaise are usually high in fat. Request that bread not be buttered, and that mayonnaise or dressing be served separately.
Meat, fish, and poultry	Choose lean cuts that are not fried, breaded, or battered. Preparation choices include roasted, baked, grilled, broiled, or boiled. Choices include lean roast beef, roast veal, small lean steak (tenderloin or sirloin), veal chop or pork chop cutlet, roast lamb, lamb chop, and poultry (remove the skin). Remove all visible fat and request that meat be served without gravy or sauce. Eat only the serving size that is part of your food plan, and take the rest home to use in another meal.
Eggs	Choose soft, hard-cooked, or poached, or request that the minimum of fat be used when scrambling or making an omelet. Request low-cholesterol eggs if you are controlling your cholesterol intake. Avoid fried or creamed eggs if you are limiting your fat intake, or avoiding saturated fat.
Fruit	Select fresh fruit or unsweetened fruit juices in portion sizes based on your food plan. Even if it is not on the menu, fresh fruit is often available.
Vegetables	Choose any vegetable prepared without sauce, butter, or margarine. Most restaurants can easily steam or microwave vegetables, if requested. Request lemon juice or vinegar to put on them if you need a little zing.
Bread	Choose plain breads and rolls, soda crackers, rye crisps, tortillas, or melba toast. Avoid rich muffins, cornbread, sweet rolls, coffee cakes, and doughnuts.

Source: Adapted from Kulkarni, K: "Adjusting nutrition therapy for special situations." In *Handbook of Diabetes Medical Nutrition Therapy,* MA Powers, Ed., Aspen Publishers, Gaithersburg, Maryland, 1996.

- Put half of a large serving in a take-home container when it is served.
- Ask for the breadbasket or extra food to be removed from the table if you are tempted to eat it.
- Avoid "all you can eat" buffets unless you can easily control how much you *do* eat.

Measuring Secrets

It can be difficult to accurately measure your food when you are away from home. The tips for estimating food portions in the following table can be quite valuable in helping you keep your food intake consistent. Try these measurements at home so you are prepared when you eat away from home.

Tips for Estimating Food Portions

Exact Measurement	Hand Measurement*	Round Object Measurement	Other Object Measurement
1 teaspoon	Tip of thumb	—	—
1 tablespoon	Whole thumb	—	—
2 tablespoons		Golf ball	
½ cup	Tight fist†	Tennis ball	
1 cup	Fist†	Baseball (hardball)	
3 oz meat	Palm of average woman's hand (no fingers or thumb)**		Deck of cards or a 3 × 5 index card
3 oz hamburger patty		Mayonnaise jar lid	
Apple or orange		Tennis ball	

*Based on a woman's hand.
†A man's fist may be 1 cup; use your fist as a guide, then actually measure the food.
**A man's hand may represent 4–6 oz of meat and that may be his serving size.

Tips for Eating at Fast-Food Restaurants

During a rushed day, going to a fast-food restaurant may be the only option for a quick meal. The problem with fast foods, however, is that they are often high in calories, fat, and sodium. Thoughtful selection is needed.

Most fast-food restaurants will provide a nutrient analysis of their food items. This information may be posted on a wall, available from someone at the service counter, on the internet, or available from the restaurant's toll-free phone number. This information will make it easier to determine what mix of foods will match your meal plan. The nutrient content of some fast foods is in appendix E.

Fast-Food Restaurant Tips

- Ask that sandwiches be made without sauces, mayonnaise, sour cream, guacamole, and cheese.
- Avoid items that are fried or battered, such as battered fish and fried chicken.
- Ask how food items are prepared if their names are confusing.
- Request extra tomato, lettuce, or salsa, if you like.
- Do not super size—choose regular or junior items.
- Fill up on salad with low-calorie dressing, if available.
- Choose low-fat milk, water, or diet soda to drink.
- Choose a baked potato over fries, if available.
- Choose baked chips over regular chips.

ALCOHOL

Drinking alcohol responsibly is important for everyone, but is especially important for people with diabetes. Alcohol is consumed at home and away from home. It is discussed in this chapter because it becomes more of a concern when you may be driving, distracted when eating at a social event, or not having ready access to food—all of which may be more likely when you are away from home.

The four primary concerns with alcohol and diabetes are:

- Alcohol consumption can cause a low-blood-glucose episode.
- Alcohol can impair memory and judgment causing someone with diabetes to skip meals and their diabetes medicine.
- Alcohol beverages typically have no nutritional value, are high in calories, and can impede weight loss or maintenance efforts.
- A low-blood-glucose episode may be confused with being "drunk" or "tipsy" if someone has been drinking alcohol. This would delay proper treatment for a low-blood-glucose episode.

Alcohol can lower blood glucose levels even after breakfast, after several drinks the previous evening. Therefore, an additional snack or a decrease in a rapid- or short-acting insulin may be necessary after you have had a drink or two. Checking your blood glucose levels will be your guide as for what you need to do. Since drinking alcohol can cause a dangerous situation, drink responsibly, wear diabetes identification, and let some other responsible person know what alcohol can do to your blood glucose. In some areas, emergency medical staff are not allowed to look in peoples' wallets or purses. Therefore, wearing a diabetes identification bracelet or necklace is important.

The carbohydrate in some alcohol beverages can raise your blood glucose, but do not rely on that to prevent a low-blood-glucose episode. You still need to eat your regular meal. Enjoying an occasional drink may be fine, but discuss this with your doctor and dietitian to see how it fits into your food plan. This is an especially important decision for young adults when they first begin to drink; learn how to do it safely.

Alcohol and carbohydrate calories you consume from these beverages can add a lot of calories to one's food plan and cause weight gain, making diabetes more difficult to care for. When you drink you can count the alcohol calories as fat calories since both are metabolized the same way.

Although someone who has diabetes should never drink on an

empty stomach, alcohol may be served prior to any food being served. You can always refuse with a gracious "I'll wait" or "No, thank you" response. Do not feel pressured to consume alcohol at any time.

Tips for Consuming Alcohol

- Drink only when diabetes is well controlled and after discussing it with your doctor.
- Do not drink if you have high triglyceride levels, are pregnant, or are planning on becoming pregnant, or you are taking certain medications (check with your pharmacist or doctor).
- Drink only with meals or snacks, never on an empty stomach.
- Limit intake to one drink per day for women and two drinks per day for men. One alcoholic drink equals:
  - 12 oz (1½ cups) of regular beer (about 150 calories)
  - 1½ oz (3 tablespoons) of liquor, such as whiskey, scotch, rum, gin, or vodka (about 100 calories)
  - 4 oz (½ cup) of wine (about 90 calories)
  - 12 oz wine cooler (high in carbohydrate about 240 calories)
- Avoid high-sugar mixes and high-carbohydrate drinks, such as daiquiri mixes, margaritas, and slow gin fizzes, as they contain sugar or syrup flavorings, juices, and regular soda. Choose water, sugar-free tonic, club soda, diet soda as mixers. One daiquiri has about 225 calories; one manhattan 260 calories; one martini 250 calories.
- Check blood glucose levels before and after drinking to see how your body reacts.
- Feel free to say "no thanks" and choose a nonalcoholic beverage.
- Wear or carry diabetes identification.
- Never drink and drive.

Alcohol and Cooking

Some foods may have alcohol (wine, sherry, liqueurs) added for flavoring. This alcohol is typically thought to evaporate, leaving the flavoring in the food. However, the cooking duration and method influences the amount of alcohol (and calories) in the food. Typically, however, the amount used is small, so any blood glucose effect or extra calories will not be significant.

Cooking wines are sometimes used in cooking instead of regular wine. These may add extra sodium to a food. The food label on the wine will give its sodium content. The range of sodium in currently available brands is 0–190 mg for every two tablespoons. This is fairly low and should not be a concern for most people. Some of the seasoned vinegars used in cooking are much higher in sodium—240 mg for every one tablespoon for a seasoned rice vinegar and 1,050 mg for every one teaspoon for a seasoned plum vinegar. You may want to ask your server if a particular food is "salty" if you are monitoring your sodium intake.

Alcohol and Heart Disease

Some studies claim that small amounts of alcohol, primarily red wine, may reduce the risk of heart disease. The reason for this is not clear. More than small amounts of alcohol (one daily glass for women and two for men), however, can lead to other health complications, and so it is not recommended that people with diabetes regularly consume alcohol. Talk to your doctor before you drink alcohol for any reason.

CHAPTER 17

Reading and Using Food Labels

One of the great advances in diabetes care happened when the food labeling regulations in the National Labeling Act took effect in 1994. Finally, you could go to the grocery store, read the food label on most foods, and immediately know the nutrient content.

No more did you have to consult a dietitian or a large nutrient analysis book to know the calories or grams of carbohydrate, fat, or sodium in one serving. Now you have this information at your fingertips to make informed decisions about your food choices—ones that ultimately affect your diabetes control.

This chapter will help you:

- Understand the three parts of a food label
- Know how to compare food labels on different food items
- Use food labels to make the best choices for you

THE THREE SECTIONS OF A FOOD LABEL

There are three main parts to a food label: the nutrition claims on the front, the nutrition facts panel, and the ingredients list.

Depending on your food plan and your health goals, you may want to use all the information or just some of it. The National Labeling Act requires information on a food label to be laid out consistently from label to label. This helps you compare one food with another to see which is a better choice for you and your diabetes. The Labeling Act carefully regulates what is permitted on a food label—the words that can be used, the size of the letters for different parts; what is mandatory information, and what is optional.

The Front of the Package

When you go to a grocery store and see all the food products, you can be overwhelmed and not know which foods are appropriate for you and your food plan. The front of a package may list features that make this product special, such as if the food helps prevent any health conditions like heart disease or tooth decay, or if the product is particularly high in a nutrient like vitamin C. Or, it may say "sugar-free," or "reduced-fat." The front of the panel tries to get you interested in the food.

Nutrition Claims

Nutrition descriptions, such as "sugar-free" and "low-fat," now have a uniform meaning from one food label to the next. See the tables and box on the following page for the rules for using various nutrition descriptions.

If a food is identified as "reduced" in calories, fat, sodium, or sugar, then that food must contain 25 percent less calories, fat, sodium, or sugar than the *regular* food.

Because you have diabetes, you may be drawn to foods that are described as "sugar-free" or "low-sugar." Even though a food may be low in sugar, it can still be high in carbohydrate. In other words, there are other ingredients in the food besides sugar that will raise your blood glucose because they contain carbohydrate. These include ingredients such as flour, cornstarch, pasta, rice, potatoes, fruit, and dried beans.

Guidelines for Using Nutrition Claims on Food Labels

Nutrient	Reduced/ Less*	Light/Lite*	Low†	Free†
Calories	25% fewer calories	33% fewer calories	40 calories or fewer	Fewer than 5 calories
Fat	25% less fat	50% less fat	3 grams or less	Less than 0.5 grams
Sodium	25% less sodium	50% less sodium	140 mg or less	Less than 5 milligrams
Sugar	25% less sugar	50% less sugar	—	Less than ½ gram

*As compared to regular, similar food.
†This is for one serving.

Guidelines for Using "Lean" and "Extra Lean" on Meat, Poultry, Seafood, and Game Meats

Lean	Extra Lean
In 3 ounces:	In 3 ounces:
• Less than 10 grams of fat	• Less than 5 grams of fat
• 4.5 grams or less saturated fat	• 2 grams or less saturated fat
• Less than 95 mg cholesterol	• Less than 95 mg cholesterol

Sugar Descriptions You May See on a Food Label

- *Sugar-free*—less than 0.5 grams of sugar per serving: other terms that can be used are *free of sugar, no sugar, zero sugar,* and *sugarless*
- *Reduced-sugar*—at least 25 percent less sugar than a regular, similar food: other terms that can be used are *less sugar* and *lower sugar*
- *No added sugar*—must contain no added sugar, such as table sugar (sucrose), milk sugar (lactose), corn sweeteners (dextrose), high-fructose corn syrup, honey, molasses, jam, jelly, and fruit juice

All of such foods can contain other carbohydrate sources and still carry one of these descriptions.

Health Claims

Health claims indicate if a food meets scientific criteria to help reduce the risk of a specific health condition. There are currently 14 health claims that are allowed on food products. Although none of them relate directly to diabetes, eight of them relate to heart disease and high blood pressure. You may want to look for these claims since heart disease and high blood pressure are prevalent in people with diabetes. Examples of such claims include:

- Limiting the amount of sodium you eat may help prevent hypertension, or high blood pressure.
- Limiting the amount of total fat you eat may help reduce your risk for some cancers.
- Limiting the amount of saturated fat and cholesterol you eat may help prevent heart disease.
- Eating high-fiber grain products, fruits, and vegetables may help prevent some cancers.
- Eating fruits, vegetables, and grain products that contain fiber may help prevent heart disease.
- Sugar alcohols do not promote tooth decay.
- Diets low in saturated fat and cholesterol that include 3 grams per day of soluble fiber from whole oats may reduce the risk of heart disease.
- Diets low in saturated fat and cholesterol that include 25 grams of soy protein a day may reduce the risk of heart disease.
- Diets low in saturated fat and cholesterol that include two servings of foods that provide a daily total of at least 3.4 grams of plant stanol esters in two meals may reduce the risk of heart disease.

Nutrition Facts Panel

The second part of the food label is the nutrition facts panel. This section gives you detailed information about the nutrients that are in one serving of the food. This information helps you decide if the food fits your needs.

On the nutrition facts panel you will see the amounts of calories, carbohydrate, protein, and fat listed as well as other information. See the illustration for a simplified nutrition facts panel. It contains the information most valuable to persons with diabetes. Depending on your needs, some information will be useful to you and other information will not. The following information must be included and is available for your use.

Nutrition Facts

Serving Size: 14 sandwiches
Servings Per Container: About 10

Amount Per Serving

Calories 160

Total Fat 8g

    Saturated Fat 1.5g

Sodium 220mg

Total Carbohydrate 18g

    Dietary Fiber 1g

Protein 3g

Simplified mini-peanut butter cracker sandwiches food label

Serving Size

Standard serving sizes are set for different types of food. For example, all cooked vegetable servings are half of a cup on food labels. This allows you to easily compare a half cup of canned kernels of corn to a half cup of canned creamed corn. One serving of juice is 1 cup, so you can compare 1 cup of orange juice to 1 cup of grape juice.

Two considerations are necessary when you use the serving size information:

- *The serving size may be different than what you normally eat.* If the label says that one serving is half of a cup and you eat 1 cup, you will be eating double the calories and other nutrients. Not only will you consume more of the vitamins and minerals, but also more calories, fat, sodium, and carbohydrate. More is not necessarily "wrong." In fact, the doubled serving size may be the right amount for your food plan.

• *The serving size may be different than a serving that is in the diabetes exchange list.* For example, the label serving size is 1 cup for fruit juice, yet in the exchange lists some juice servings are half of a cup and others are one-third of a cup. You may need help adjusting the serving size so it fits your food plan. Ask your diabetes team for help to be sure the serving sizes fit your food plan.

Calories

The number of calories listed on the nutrition facts panel is the number of calories in one serving of the food. When comparing food labels, you may want to find a food that allows you to eat a larger serving for fewer calories. For example, when you compare plain canned corn to creamed canned corn, you will find that the plain corn has about 30 fewer calories and 8 grams less of carbohydrate for the same serving size.

Nutrient Amounts

Each food label must list the amount of 11 nutrients: fat, saturated fat, cholesterol, total carbohydrate, fiber, sugars, protein, vitamin A, vitamin C, calcium, and iron. Other nutrients may be listed but are not required.

Your body needs all of the nutrients listed, but you will not need to be concerned about all of them on a daily basis. In fact, you may only want to look at one of the nutrients. Your interest will depend on your health needs and the type of food plan you are following. Use the information that you need and don't let the other information distract you.

For example, if you are counting grams (g) of carbohydrate, you would then use the number of grams on the "total carbohydrate" line as seen in the food label in the previous illustration. Total carbohydrate includes all sugar, starch, fiber, and sugar alcohol that is in one serving. Or, if you were counting grams of fat, you would use the number of fat grams on the "total fat" line.

% Daily Value

The % Daily Value compares the amount of a nutrient to what an average person needs to eat on a daily basis if he or she consumes 2,000 calories. Ideally you want to consume the recommended amount of food so you can meet or exceed the % Daily Value for beneficial nutrients, like fiber, and not exceed the % Daily Value for nutrients you may want to limit, like sodium.

Many people with diabetes consume fewer than 2,000 calories, so their daily needs may be different than those who consume 2,000 calories a day. However, some Daily Values are the same no matter how many calories you consume. The following table can help you adjust the % Daily Value goals to your calorie intake.

The Daily Value Amounts for Various Calorie Levels*

Nutrient		Calorie Level				
		1,200	1,500	1,800	2,000	2,500
Total fat grams	Less than:	40	50	60	65	80
Saturated fat (grams)	Less than:	13	16	20	20	25
Cholesterol (mg)	Less than:	300	300	300	300	300
Sodium (mg)	Less than:	2,400	2,400	2,400	2,400	2,400
Total carbohydrate (grams)		180	225	270	300	375
Dietary fiber (grams)		20	20	21	25	30

*Your daily values may vary from these amounts. The amount is based on each individual's food preferences, other health conditions, diabetes treatment, and diabetes control. Talk to your dietitian about appropriate amounts for you.

Source: Adapted from Leontos, C: *What to Eat When You Get Diabetes.* John Wiley & Sons, Inc., New York, 2000.

The Ingredients List

The third section of a food label is the ingredients list. The ingredients are listed according to the amount used in that food product. For example, the ingredients for raisin bread would list flour first and raisins later in the list. This information is useful if you have a food allergy or food intolerance, or if you want to avoid a certain ingredient.

If you have a peanut, wheat, or other food allergy you must always read the ingredient list. Because of the critical nature of food allergies and food intolerances, food companies take great care in including all ingredients, even very small amounts, in this list.

A food label contains very valuable information for people with diabetes. With the food labeling regulations that were established in the 1990s the information is now presented in a consistent manner that allows you to compare different foods. This helps you be knowledgeable and in control of the food you choose. Use the information that is most valuable to you in meeting your food plan goals. Often, people with diabetes rely on the calorie, total carbohydrate, total fat, and sodium content of a food to decide if and how a food fits their food plans.

Appendixes

APPENDIX A

Finding a Nutrition Expert and Other Diabetes Resources

This book is filled with information about diabetes and food. Yet the more you learn, the more you will want to know about other areas of diabetes as well as more in-depth information about some of the topics covered here. The following resources are great places to start your search. There are plenty of additional resources and support organizations—probably right in your own community.

A registered dietitian (RD) can help you with a food plan that meets your diabetes goals. To locate a dietitian in your area:

- Ask your doctor for a referral.
- Ask a member of your diabetes support group for suggestions.
- Call your local hospital's nutrition department. They may offer outpatient counseling and classes, or know of a dietitian who has a private practice.
- Check the yellow pages under nutrition, nutritionist, dietitian, and health.
- Contact your state or local dietetic association.
- Contact the American Dietetic Association's referral phone line or website. On the internet, go to the home page and click "Find a dietitian, your link to top food and nutrition experts." You can

request a referral for a specific topic (like diabetes) and for a specific location (by your town or your zip code, and how many miles from either).

American Dietetic Association
Phone: 1-800-366-1655
www.eatright.org

American Association of Diabetes Educators
Phone: 1-800-338-3633
www.aadenet.org

American Diabetes Association
Phone: 1-800-DIABETES (342-2383)
www.diabetes.org

Canadian Diabetes Association
Phone: 1-800-BANTING (226-8464)
www.diabetes.ca

OTHER SOURCES FOR DIABETES INFORMATION

Centers for Disease Control and Prevention, Division of Diabetes Translation

Phone: Toll-free 1-877-CDC-DIAB (232-3422)
www.cdc.gov/diabetes

Juvenile Diabetes Research Foundation International

Phone: 1-800-533-CURE (2873) or 212-785-9500
www.jdfcure.org

NATIONAL INSTITUTES OF HEALTH

National Diabetes Education Program (NDEP)

Phone: 1-800-438-5383
ndep.nih.gov

National Diabetes Information Clearinghouse (NDIC)

Phone: 1-800-860-8747 or 1-301-654-3327
www.niddk.nih.gov/health/diabetes/ndic.htm

Preventing Type 2 Diabetes

Although this book is for people who have diabetes, you may be interested in the latest research about *preventing* type 2 diabetes. You can share this information with your family and friends, and others who may be at risk for developing diabetes. We currently do not know how to prevent type 1 diabetes, so this appendix will focus just on type 2 diabetes.

WHO'S AT RISK FOR DEVELOPING TYPE 2 DIABETES?

You are at high risk for developing diabetes if you can answer yes to two or more of these questions:

- Are you 45 years old or older?
- Are you 20 pounds or more overweight?
- Do you have a parent, brother, or sister with diabetes?
- Is your family background African American, American Indian, Asian American, Hispanic, or Pacific Islander?
- Do you have high blood cholesterol or triglycerides (blood fats)?
- Do you have high blood pressure?

- Do you exercise little or not at all during a normal day?
- Do you have a history of diabetes during pregnancy?

Talk to your doctor if you are at risk so you can be checked further for diabetes. The sooner diabetes is diagnosed the sooner you can take action to help control it.

HOW TO PREVENT TYPE 2 DIABETES

If you don't have diabetes, but are at risk for developing it, there are three steps you can take to prevent it or delay its onset. This information is based on a recent study that clearly shows how to prevent diabetes when you are at risk. Almost 60% of those at risk for developing type 2 diabetes were able to prevent it in this study. This is great news! And here are the three steps:

1. Be physically active at least 30 minutes per day.
2. Lose 5–7% of your body weight.
3. Learn about and make lifestyle choices and get ongoing support.

Type 2 diabetes takes time to develop and may begin 10–15 years before you are diagnosed. It does not happen overnight. If you are at risk for developing diabetes, start now with these steps to prevent diabetes or delay its onset. Once you get diabetes you need to be more careful with what you eat (how much food and when), you need to be physically active, and you may need medication to help control your blood sugar. This book explains all the steps to control diabetes and you can do that, but it is much easier to take these three steps to prevent or delay diabetes.

Be Physically Active

Most people in the research group who did not get diabetes during the study were physically active for at least 30 minutes almost every day. Usually the activity was walking, but other moderate intensity activities were also done. This recommendation, to be active at least 30 minutes on five or more days a week, is lower than the new recommendation (60 minutes each day) from the National Academy of Sciences. So begin now when you have the possibility of preventing or delaying diabetes. Then you can gradually increase your time.

Lose Weight

Losing a little bit of weight has a dramatic effect on how your body uses its insulin. In this study, those who were able to prevent diabetes lost as little as 5–7% of their body weight. To get an idea of how much this is, consider someone who weighs 175 pounds. He or she would need to lose 9 to 12 pounds. Someone who weighs 225 pounds would need to lose 11 to 16 pounds. For most people, this is not a huge weight loss and can be maintained with reasonable changes in food intake and activity.

Make Lifestyle Choices

In addition, each person who was selected to get the more intensive treatment in the study had 16 individual or group sessions to learn about making the best eating and activity choices. After the 16 sessions, follow-up was once a month. This was a critical component of the study as each participant learned what he or she could personally do to make changes and to make those changes part of their life. They also learned what parts of their lifestyle were already healthy so they could continue making those choices. The support and information from the health care providers obviously was necessary, so don't miss this component of the prevention plan!

EXAMINING THE RESEARCH

This guidance on diabetes prevention is based upon the findings of the Diabetes Prevention Program (DPP) sponsored by the National

Institutes of Health. Over 3,000 people participated in the DPP. They were all overweight, had an average age of 51 years, and had some higher than ideal levels of blood sugar (impaired glucose tolerance) but not high enough to be diagnosed with diabetes. About half of the participants were African American, American Indian, Asian American, Pacific Islander, or Hispanic.

The study ended early because the results were so clear–type 2 diabetes could be prevented with some lifestyle changes.

Another prevention study also showed that lifestyle changes could prevent type 2 diabetes. The acclaimed Finnish Diabetes Prevention Study showed a similar decrease in type 2 diabetes when participants lost weight, followed a low-saturated-fat, higher-fiber diet, increased physical activity, and saw a nutritionist seven times the first year and four times a year in following years.

Two other studies identified a particular type of food to help reduce diabetes risk. The Harvard Nurses Health Study and the Iowa Women's Health Study found that study participants who ate the most whole-grain foods had a lower risk of developing type 2 diabetes. Another recent study concluded that whole grains decrease heart disease in a number of ways. Whole grains help reduce cholesterol levels and reduce blood pressure. Whole grains also help your body use insulin better and improve blood glucose control. It seems very clear that whole grain foods are important to eat when you are at risk for developing diabetes (have pre-diabetes) and when you have diabetes.

These are just a few of the studies that showed that healthy eating, moderate weight loss, and regular physical activity can reduce the risk of diabetes. It is clear that if you are at risk for type 2 diabetes, you can take action to help prevent or delay the onset of diabetes.

TAKING ACTION

If you are at risk for diabetes, take action now. Don't delay, as it may take you awhile to work up to 30–60 minutes of activity a day and lose some weight. Start gradually with small changes that are doable for you.

Also talk to others who may be at risk. You may want to start a group that meets occasionally for additional support and ideas. The National Institutes of Health publication titled *Am I at Risk for Type 2 Diabetes?* offers additional information that you can read on the internet at www.niddk.nih.gov under "Health Information" or you can order by calling 1-800-860-8747.

To get started:

- Talk to your doctor about your diabetes risk factors and what you can do about them.
- Set up an appointment with a dietitian to improve your eating habits.
- Keep track of physical activity for a week so you know how active you are right now and gradually become more active until you do at least 30 minutes of moderate activity five or more days a week.
- Talk to your family about changes you can make together to prevent or delay diabetes.

APPENDIX C

Your Food Diary

		Today's Date: _____
Time	Blood Glucose/ Meds	Everything I Ate and Drank Today and How Much

Today's Activity and Notes:

APPENDIX D

Food Exchange Lists

A s you read in chapter 15, exchange lists are foods listed together because they are alike. Each food serving has about the same amount of carbohydrate, protein, fat, and calories as the other foods on that list. This is the reason any food on a list can be "exchanged" or traded for any other food on the same list.

The exchange lists give you many food choices. Several foods, such as beans, peas, lentils, bacon, and peanut butter, are on two lists. This adds flexibility in putting together meals. Whenever choosing new foods or varying your meal plan, monitor your blood glucose to see how these different foods affect your blood glucose level.

STARCH LIST

One starch exchange equals 15 grams of carbohydrate, 3 grams of protein, 0–1 grams of fat, and 80 calories per serving.

Starch	One Exchange/ Serving
Bread	
Bagel (varies), 4 oz	¼ (1 oz)
Bread (white, pumpernickel, whole wheat, rye)	1 slice

(continued)

(continued)
Starch

	One Exchange/ Serving
Bread, reduced calorie or "lite"	2 slices
Bread sticks, crisp, 4 in. long × ½ in.	2 (⅔ oz)
English muffin	½
Hot dog or hamburger bun	½ (1 oz)
Muffin, 5 oz	⅕ (1 oz)
Pancake, 4 in. across, 1⁄4 in. thick	1
Pita, 6 in. across	½
Raisin bread, unfrosted	1 slice (1 oz)
Tortilla, corn, 6 in. across	1
Tortilla, flour, 6 in. across	1
Tortilla, flour, 10 in. across	⅓
Waffle, 4 in. square or across, reduced-fat	1

Cereals and Grains

Barley or couscous	⅓ cup
Bran cereals	½ cup
Bulgur	½ cup
Cereals, cooked	½ cup
Cereals, unsweetened, ready-to-eat	¾ cup
Cornmeal (dry)	3 Tbsp
Flour (dry)	3 Tbsp
Granola, low-fat	¼ cup
Grape-Nuts	¼ cup
Grits	½ cup
Kasha	½ cup
Millet	¼ cup
Muesli	¼ cup
Oats	½ cup
Pasta	⅓ cup
Puffed cereal	1½ cups
Rice, white or brown	⅓ cup
Shredded Wheat	½ cup
Sugar-frosted cereal	½ cup
Wheat germ	3 Tbsp

Starchy Vegetables

Baked beans	⅓ cup

Starch	One Exchange/ Serving
Corn	½ cup
Corn on the cob, large	½ cob (5 oz)
Corn on the cob, medium	1 (5 oz)
Mixed vegetables with corn, peas, or pasta	1 cup
Peas, green	½ cup
Plantain	½ cup
Potato, baked with skin	¼ large (3 oz)
Potato, boiled	½ cup or ½ medium (3 oz)
Squash, winter (acorn, butternut, pumpkin)	1 cup
Yam, sweet potato, plain	½ cup

Crackers and Snacks

Animal crackers	8
Graham crackers, 2½ in. square	3
Matzoh	¾ oz
Melba toast	4 slices
Oyster crackers	24
Popcorn (popped, no fat added or low-fat microwave)	3 cups
Pretzels	¾ oz
Rice cakes, 4 in. across	2
Saltine-type crackers	6
Snack chips, fat-free (tortilla, potato)	15–20 (¾ oz)
Whole-wheat crackers, no fat added	2–5 (¾ oz)

Beans, Peas, and Lentils
(Count as one starch exchange, plus one very lean meat exchange.)

Beans and peas (garbanzo, pinto, kidney, white, split, black-eyed)	½ cup
Lima beans	⅔ cup
Lentils	½ cup
Miso*	3 Tbsp

Starchy Foods Prepared with Fat
(Count as one starch exchange, plus one fat exchange.)

Biscuit, 2½ in. across	1
Chow mein noodles	½ cup
Corn bread, 2 in. cube	1 (2 oz)
Crackers, round butter type	6

(continued)

(continued) Starch	One Exchange/ Serving
Croutons	1 cup
French-fried potatoes (oven baked)	1 cup (2 oz)
Granola	¼ cup
Hummus	⅓ cup
Popcorn, microwave	3 cups
Sandwich cracker, cheese or peanut butter filling	3
Snack chips (potato, tortilla)	9–13 (¾ oz)
Stuffing, bread (prepared)	⅓ cup
Taco shell, 6 in. across	2
Waffle, 4 in. square	1
Whole-wheat crackers, fat added	4–6 (1 oz)

*400 mg or more sodium per exchange

FRUIT LIST

One fruit exchange equals 15 grams of carbohydrate, and 60 calories per serving. The weight includes skin, core, seeds, and rind.

Fruit	One Exchange/ Serving
Apple, unpeeled, small	1 (4 oz)
Applesauce, unsweetened	½ cup
Apples, dried	4 rings
Apricots, fresh	4 whole (5½ oz)
Apricots, dried	8 halves
Apricots, canned	½ cup
Banana, small	1 (4 oz)
Blackberries	¾ cup
Blueberries	¾ cup
Cantaloupe, small	⅓ melon (11 oz) or 1 cup cubes
Cherries, sweet, fresh	12 (3 oz)
Cherries, sweet, canned	½ cup
Dates	3
Figs, fresh	1½ large or 2 medium (3½ oz)

Fruit	One Exchange/ Serving
Figs, dried	1½
Fruit cocktail	½ cup
Grapefruit, large	½ (11 oz)
Grapefruit sections, canned	¾ cup
Grapes, small	17 (3 oz)
Honeydew melon	1 slice (10 oz) or 1 cup cubes
Kiwi	1 (3½ oz)
Mandarin oranges, canned	¾ cup
Mango, small	½ fruit (5½ oz) or ½ cup
Nectarine, small	1 (5 oz)
Orange, small	1 (6½ oz)
Papaya	½ fruit (8 oz) or 1 cup cubes
Peach, medium, fresh	1 (6 oz)
Peaches, canned	½ cup
Pear, large, fresh	½ (4 oz)
Pears, canned	½ cup
Pineapple, fresh	¾ cup
Pineapple, canned	½ cup
Plums, small	2 (5 oz)
Plums, canned	½ cup
Plums, dried (prunes)	3
Raisins	2 Tbsp
Raspberries	1 cup
Strawberries	1¼ cup whole berries
Tangerines, small	2 (8 oz)
Watermelon	1 slice (13½ oz) or 1½ cup cubes

Fruit Juice

Apple juice/cider	½ cup
Cranberry juice cocktail	⅓ cup
Cranberry juice cocktail, reduced-calorie	1 cup
Fruit juice blends, 100% juice	⅓ cup

(continued)

(continued) Fruit	One Exchange/ Serving
Grape juice	⅓ cup
Grapefruit juice	½ cup
Orange juice	⅓ cup
Pineapple juice	½ cup
Prune juice	⅓ cup

MILK LIST

One milk exchange equals 12 grams of carbohydrate and 8 grams protein.

Milk	One Exchange/ Serving
Fat-Free and Low-Fat Milk (0–3 grams fat per serving)	
Fat-free milk	1 cup
0.5% milk	1 cup
1% milk	1 cup
Fat-free or low-fat buttermilk	1 cup
Evaporated fat-free milk	½ cup
Fat-free dry milk	⅓ cup dry
Yogurt, plain, fat-free	⅔ cup (6 oz)
Yogurt, fat-free, sweetened with nonnutritive sweetener and fructose	⅔ cup (6 oz)
Soy milk, low-fat/fat-free	1 cup
Reduced fat (5 grams fat per serving)	
2% milk	1 cup
Soy milk	1 cup
Sweet acidophilus milk	1 cup
Yogurt, plain low-fat	¾ cup
Whole Milk (8 grams fat per serving)	
Whole milk	1 cup
Evaporated whole milk	½ cup

Milk	One Exchange/ Serving
Goat's milk	1 cup
Kefir	1 cup
Yogurt, plain (made from whole milk)	¾ cut

SWEETS, DESSERTS, AND OTHER CARBOHYDRATES LIST

One exchange in this list equals 15 grams carbohydrates, or 1 starch, or 1 fruit, or 1 milk.

Carbohydrate	Serving Size	Exchanges per Serving
Angel food cake, unfrosted	1/12 cake (about 2 oz)	2 carbs
Brownie, small, unfrosted	2 in. square (about 1 oz)	1 carb, 1 fat
Cake, unfrosted	2 in. square (about 1 oz)	1 carb, 1 fat
Cake, frosted	2 in. square (about 2 oz)	2 carbs, 1 fat
Cookie or sandwich cookie with crème filling	2 small (about ⅔ oz)	1 carb, 1 fat
Cookies, sugar-free	3 small or 1 large (¾–1 oz)	1 carb, 1–2 fat
Cranberry sauce, jellied	¼ cup	1½ carbs
Cupcake, frosted	1 small (about 2 oz)	2 carbs, 1 fat
Doughnut, plain cake	1 medium (1½oz)	1½ carbs, 2 fats
Doughnut, glazed	3¾ in. across (2 oz)	2 carbs, 2 fats
Energy, sport, or breakfast bar	1 bar (1⅓ oz)	1½ carbs, 0–1 fat
Energy, sport, or breakfast bar	1 bar (2 oz)	2 carbs, 1 fat
Fruit juice bars, frozen, 100% juice	1 bar (3 oz)	1 carb
Fruit snacks, chewy (pureed fruit concentrate)	1 roll (¾ oz)	1 carb
Fruit spreads, 100% fruit	1½ Tbsp	1 carb
Gelatin, regular	½ cup	1 carb
Gingersnaps	3	1 carb
Granola or snack bar, regular or low-fat	1 bar (1 oz)	1½ carbs
Honey	1 Tbsp	1 carb

(continued)

(continued) Carbohydrate	Serving Size	Exchanges per Serving
Ice cream	½ cup	1 carb, 2 fats
Ice cream, light	½ cup	1 carb, 1 fat
Ice cream, low-fat	½ cup	1½ carbs
Ice cream, fat-free, no sugar added	½ cup	1 carb
Jam or jelly, regular	1 Tbsp	1 carb
Reduced calorie meal replacement shake	1 can (10–11 oz)	1½ carbs, 0–1 fat
Milk, chocolate, whole	1 cup	2 carbs, 1 fat
Pie, fruit, 2 crusts	⅙ pie	3 carbs, 2 fats
Pie, pumpkin or custard	⅛ pie	2 carbs, 2 fats
Pudding, regular (made with reduced-fat milk)	½ cup	2 carbs
Pudding, sugar-free (made with low-fat milk)	½ cup	1 carb
Pudding, sugar-free or sugar-free and fat-free (made with fat-free milk)	½ cup	1 carb
Rice milk, fat-free or low-fat plain	1 cup	1 carb
Rice milk, low-fat, flavored	1 cup	1½ carbs
Salad dressing, fat-free*	¼ cup	1 carb
Sherbet, sorbet	½ cup	2 carbs
Spaghetti or pasta sauce canned*	½ cup	1 carb, 1 fat
Sports drink	8 oz (about 1 cup)	1 carb
Sugar	1 Tbsp	1 carb
Sweet roll or Danish	1 (2½ oz)	2½ carbs, 2 fats
Syrup, light	2 Tbsp	1 carb
Syrup, regular	1 Tbsp	1 carb
Syrup, regular	¼ cup	4 carbs
Vanilla wafers	5	1 carb, 1 fat
Yogurt, frozen	½ cup	1 carb, 0–1 fat
Yogurt, frozen, low-fat	⅓ cup	1 carb, 0–1 fat
Yogurt, frozen, fat-free	⅓ cup	1 carb
Yogurt, low-fat with fruit	1 cup	3 carbs, 0–1 fat

*400 mg or more sodium per exchange

NONSTARCHY VEGETABLE LIST

One vegetable exchange is ½ cup of cooked vegetables or vegetable juice, or 1 cup of raw vegetables. One vegetable exchange equals 5 grams carbohydrate, 2 grams protein, 0 grams fat, and 25 calories.

Vegetable
Artichoke
Artichoke hearts
Asparagus
Beans (green, wax, Italian)
Bean sprouts
Beets
Broccoli
Brussels sprouts
Cabbage
Carrots
Cauliflower
Celery
Cucumber
Eggplant
Green onions or scallions
Greens (collard, kale, mustard, turnip)
Kohlrabi
Leeks
Mixed vegetables (without corn, peas, or pasta)
Mushrooms
Okra
Onions
Pea pods
Pepper (all varieties)
Radishes
Salad greens (endive, escarole, lettuce, romaine, spinach)
Sauerkraut*
Spinach
Summer squash

Tomato
Tomatoes, canned
Tomato sauce*
Tomato/vegetable juice*
Turnips
Water chestnuts
Watercress
Zucchini

*400 mg or more sodium per exchange

MEAT AND MEAT SUBSTITUTES LIST

Very Lean Meat and Substitutes List

One exchange equals 0 grams carbohydrate, 7 grams protein, 0–1 grams fat, and 35 calories.

One very lean meat exchange is equal to any one of the following items:

Meat	One Exchange/ Serving
Poultry: Chicken or turkey (white meat, no skin), Cornish hen (no skin)	1 oz
Fish: Fresh or frozen cod, flounder, haddock, halibut, trout; tuna (fresh or canned in water)	1 oz
Shellfish: Clams, crab, lobster, scallops, shrimp, imitation shellfish	1 oz
Game Duck or pheasant (no skin), venison, buffalo, ostrich	1 oz
Cheese with 1 gram or less fat per ounce:	
Nonfat or low-fat cottage cheese	¼ cup
Fat-free cheese	1 oz
Fat-free or low-fat cottage cheese	¼ cup
Other: Processed sandwich meats with 1 gram or less fat per ounce, such as deli-thin shaved meats, chipped beef*, turkey ham	1 oz
Egg whites	2
Egg substitutes, plain	¼ cup
Hot dogs with 1 gram or less fat per ounce*	1 oz

Meat	One Exchange/ Serving
Kidney (high in cholesterol)	1 oz
Sausage with 1 gram or less fat per ounce	1 oz
Beans, peas, lentils (cooked) (Count as one very lean meat and one starch exchange.)	½ cup

*400 mg or more sodium per exchange

Lean Meat and Substitutes List

One exchange equals 0 grams carbohydrate, 7 grams protein, 3 grams fat, and 55 calories.

One lean meat exchange is equal to any one of the following items:

Meat	One Exchange/ Serving
Beef: USDA Select or Choice grades of lean beef trimmed of fat, such as round, sirloin, and flank steak; tenderloin; roast (rib, chuck, rump); steak (T-bone, porterhouse, cubed), ground round	1 oz
Pork: Lean pork, such as fresh ham; canned, cured, or boiled ham; Canadian bacon*; tenderloin, center loin chop	1 oz
Lamb: Roast, chop, leg	1 oz
Veal: Lean chop, roast	1 oz
Poultry: Chicken, turkey (dark meat, no skin), chicken (white meat, with skin), domestic duck or goose (well drained of fat, no skin)	1 oz
Fish:	
Herring (uncreamed or smoked)	1 oz
Oysters	6 medium
Salmon (fresh or canned), catfish	1 oz
Sardines (canned)	2 medium
Tuna (canned in oil, drained)	1 oz
Game: Goose (no skin), rabbit	1 oz
Cheese:	
4.5%-fat cottage cheese	¼ cup
Grated Parmesan	2 Tbsp
Cheeses with 3 grams or less fat per ounce	1 oz
Other:	
Hot dogs with 3 grams or less fat per ounce*	1½ oz

(continued)

(continued) **Meat**	**One Exchange/** **Serving**
Other (continued): Processed sandwich meat with 3 grams or less fat per ounce, such as turkey pastrami or kielbasa Liver, heart (high in cholesterol) Tofu, light	 1 oz 1 oz ½ cup or 4 oz

*400 mg or more sodium per exchange

Medium-Fat Meat and Substitutes List

One exchange equals 0 grams carbohydrate, 7 grams protein, 5 grams fat, 75 calories.

One medium-fat meat exchange is equal to any one of the following items:

Meat	**One Exchange/** **Serving**
Beef: Most beef products fall into this category (ground beef; meatloaf; corned beef; short ribs; prime grades of meat trimmed of fat, such as prime rib)	1 oz
Pork: Top loin, chop Boston butt, cutlet	1 oz
Lamb: Rib roast, ground	1 oz
Veal: Cutlet (ground or cubed, unbreaded)	1 oz
Poultry: Chicken (dark meat, with skin), ground turkey or ground chicken, fried chicken (with skin)	1 oz
Fish: Any fried fish product	1 oz
Cheese with 5 grams or less fat per ounce: Feta Mozzarella Ricotta	 1 oz 1 oz ¼ cup (2 oz)
Other: Egg (high in cholesterol, limit to 3 per week) Sausage with 5 grams or less fat per ounce Tempeh Tofu	 1 1 oz ¼ cup 4 oz or ½ cup

High-Fat Meat and Substitutes List

One exchange equals 0 grams carbohydrate, 7 grams protein, 8 grams fat, and 100 calories. Remember these items are high in saturated fat, cholesterol, and calories and may raise blood cholesterol levels if eaten on a regular basis.

One high-fat meat exchange is equal to any of the following items.

Meat	One Exchange/ Serving
Pork: Spareribs, ground pork, pork sausage	1 oz
Cheese: All regular cheeses, such as American*, cheddar, Monterey Jack, Swiss	1 oz
Other:	
Processed sandwich meat with 8 grams or less fat per ounce, such as bologna, pimento loaf, salami	1 oz
Sausage, such as bratwurst, Italian knockwurst, Polish, smoked	1 oz
Hot dog (turkey or chicken)*	1 (10/lb)
Bacon	3 slices (20 slices/lb)
Hot dog* (beef, pork, or combination) (Count as one high-fat meat plus one fat exchange.)	1 (10/lb)
Peanut butter (contains unsaturated fat)	1 Tbsp

*400 mg or more sodium per exchange

FAT LIST

Fat	One Exchange/ Serving
Monosaturated Fats (One fat exchange equals 5 grams of fat and 45 calories.)	
Avocado, medium	2 Tbsp (1 oz)
Oil (canola, olive, peanut)	1 tsp
Olives, ripe (black)	8 large
Olives, green, stuffed*	10 large
Nuts	
Almonds, cashews	6 nuts
Mixed (50% peanuts)	6 nuts
Peanuts	10 nuts
Pecans	4 halves
Peanut butter, smooth or crunchy	2 tsp
Sesame seeds	1 Tbsp
Tahini paste	2 tsp

(continued)

(continued) **Fat**	**One Exchange/ Serving**
Polyunsaturated Fats (One fat exchange equals 5 grams and 45 calories.)	
Margarine, stick, tub, or squeeze	1 tsp
Margarine, lower-fat spread (30%–50% vegetable oil)	1 Tbsp
Mayonnaise, regular	1 tsp
Mayonnaise, reduced-fat	1 Tbsp
Nuts, walnuts, English	4 halves
Oil (corn, safflower, soybean)	1 tsp
Salad dressing, regular*	1 Tbsp
Salad dressing, reduced-fat	2 Tbsp
Miracle Whip Salad Dressing, regular	2 tsp
Miracle Whip Salad Dressing, reduced-fat	1 Tbsp
Seeds (pumpkin, sunflower)	1 Tbsp
Saturated Fats** (One fat exchange equals 5 grams of fat and 45 calories.)	
Bacon, cooked	1 slice (20 slices/lb)
Bacon, grease	1 tsp
Butter, stick	1 tsp
Butter, whipped	2 tsp
Butter, reduced-fat	1 Tbsp
Chitterlings, boiled	2 Tbsp (½ oz)
Coconut, sweetened, shredded	2 Tbsp
Cream, half and half	2 Tbsp
Cream cheese, regular	1 Tbsp (½ oz)
Cream cheese, reduced-fat	1½ Tbsp (¾ oz)
Fatback or salt pork†	
Shortening or lard	1 tsp
Sour cream, regular	2 Tbsp
Sour cream reduced-fat	3 Tbsp

*400 mg or more sodium per exchange.

†Use a piece 1 in. × 1 in. × ¼ in. if you plan to eat the fatback cooked with vegetables. Use a piece 2 in. × 1 in. × ½ in. when eating only the vegetables with the fatback removed.

**Saturated fats can raise blood cholesterol levels.

FREE FOODS LIST

A free food is any food or drink that contains less than 20 calories or less than 5 grams of carb per serving. Foods with a serving size listed should be limited to three servings per day. Be sure to spread them out throughout the day. Foods listed without a serving size can be eaten as often as you like.

Starch	One Exchange/ Serving
Fat-Free or Reduced-Fat Foods	
Cream cheese, fat-free	1 Tbsp (½ oz)
Creamers, nondairy, liquid	1 Tbsp
Creamers, nondairy, powdered	2 tsp
Mayonnaise, fat-free	1 Tbsp
Mayonnaise, reduced-fat	1 tsp
Margarine spread, fat-free	4 Tbsp
Margarine spread, reduced-fat	1 tsp
Miracle Whip, fat-free	1 Tbsp
Miracle Whip, reduced-fat	1 tsp
Nonstick cooking spray	
Salad dressing, fat-free or low-fat	1 Tbsp
Salad dressing, fat-free Italian	2 Tbsp
Sour cream, fat-free, reduced-fat	1 Tbsp
Whipped topping, regular	1 Tbsp
Whipped topping, light or fat free	2 Tbsp
Sugar-free Foods	
Candy, hard, sugar-free	1 candy
Gelatin dessert, sugar-free	
Gelatin, unflavored	
Gum, sugar-free	
Jam or jelly, light	2 tsp
Sugar substitutes*	
Syrup, sugar-free	2 Tbsp
Drinks	
Bouillon, broth, consommé†	
Bouillon or broth, low-sodium	
Carbonated or mineral water	

(continued)

(continued) Starch	One Exchange/ Serving
Club soda	
Cocoa powder, unsweetened	1 Tbsp
Coffee	
Diet soft drinks, sugar-free	
Drink mixes, sugar-free	
Tea	
Tonic water, sugar-free	

Condiments	
Ketchup	1 Tbsp
Horseradish	
Lemon juice	
Lime juice	
Mustard	
Pickles, dill†	1½ large
Salsa	¼ cup
Soy sauce, regular or light†	
Taco sauce	1 Tbsp
Vinegar	

Seasonings**	
Flavoring extracts	
Garlic	
Herbs, fresh or dried	
Pimento	
Spices	
Tabasco or hot pepper sauce	
Wine, used in cooking	
Worcestershire sauce	

*Sugar substitutes, alternatives, or replacements that are approved by the Food and Drug Administration (FDA) are safe to use. Common brand names include Equal (aspartame), Splenda (sucralose), Sprinkle Sweet (saccharin), Sweet One (acesulfame K), Sweet-10 (saccharin), Sugar Twin (saccharin), and Sweet 'n Low (saccharin).

†400 mg or more sodium per exchange.

**Be careful with seasonings that contain sodium or are salts, such as garlic or celery salt, and lemon pepper.

COMBINATION FOODS LIST

Following are exchanges for typical combination foods. Ask your dietitian for information about other combination foods you would like to eat.

Food	Serving Size	Exchanges per Serving
Entrees		
Tuna noodle casserole, lasagna, spaghetti with meatballs, chili with beans, macaroni with cheese*	1 cup (8 oz)	2 carbs, 2 medium fat meats
Chow mein (without noodles, rice)*	2 cups (16 oz)	1 carb, 2 lean meats
Frozen entrees and meals		
Dinner-type meal	generally 14–17 oz	3 carbs, 3 medium-fat meats, 3 fats
Meatless burger, soy based	3 oz	½ carb, 1 lean meat
Meatless burger, vegetable and starch based	3 oz	1 carb, 1 lean meat
Pizza, cheese, thin crust*	¼ of 10 In (5 oz)	2 carbs, 2 medium-fat meats, 1 fat
Pizza, meat topping, thin crust*	¼ of 10 in. (5 oz)	2 carbs, 2 medium-fat meats, 2 fats
Pot pie*	1 (7 oz)	2½ carbs, 1 medium-fat meat, 3 fats
Entrée with less than 400 calories*	1 (11 oz)	2–3 carbs, 1–2 lean meats
Soups		
Bean*	1 cup	1 carb, 1 very lean meat
Cream (made with water)*	1 cup (8 oz)	1 carb, 1 fat
Instant*	6 oz prepared	1 carb
Instant with beans or lentils*	8 oz prepared	2½ carbs, 1 very lean meat

(continued)

(continued) Food	Serving Size	Exchanges per Serving
Split soup (made with water)*	½ cup (4 oz)	1 carb
Tomato (made with water)*	1 cup (8 oz)	1 carb
Vegetable beef, chicken noodle, or other broth-type*	1 cup (8 oz)	1 carb

*400 mg or more sodium per exchange

Source: ©2003, *Exchange Lists for Meal Planning.* American Dietetic Association and American Diabetes Association, Chicago, Illinois, 2003; used with permission.

Fast Food Restaurant Guide

E ating at a *fast* food restaurant may be very convenient, but be aware that calories and carbohydrates also add up *fast*. The following will help you know how some of these foods fit into your food plan. (Note that all information is correct as of this writing.) Contact these restaurants, and other restaurants, for information on additional foods. You may also want to check on the sodium and saturated fat content of the foods.

Burger King

Food	Size	Calories	Carbohydrate (grams)	Exchanges
Big King Sandwich	1	640	28	2 carb, 5 medium-fat meat, 3 fat
BK Broiler Chicken	1	530	45	3 carb, 3 medium-fat meat, 2 fat
BK Big Fish	1	720	59	4 carb, 2 medium-fat meat, 7 fat
Hamburger	1	320	27	2 carb, 2 medium-fat meat, 1 fat
Whopper	1	660	47	3 carb, 3 medium-fat meat, 5 fat

(continued)

245

(continued)

Food	Size	Calories	Carbohydrate (grams)	Exchanges
Chicken Tenders	5 pieces	230	11	1 carb, 2 medium-fat meat, 1 fat
Onion Rings	1 medium order	380	46	3 carb, 4 fat
Shake, Vanilla	1 medium	430	73	5 carb, 2 fat

McDonald's

Food	Size	Calories	Carbohydrate (grams)	Exchanges
Big Mac	1	560	45	3 carb, 2 medium-fat meat, 4 fat
Filet-O-Fish	1	450	42	3 carb, 1 medium-fat meat, 4 fat
French Fries	1 small order	210	26	2 carb, 2 fat
French Fries	1 super-sized	540	68	4½ carb, 5 fat
Egg McMuffin (sausage/egg)	1	440	27	2 carb, 2 medium-fat meat, 4 fat
Low-Fat Apple Bran Muffin	1	300	61	4 carb, 1 fat
Ice Cream Cone, Reduced-Fat Vanilla	1	150	23	1½ carb, 1 fat
M&M McFlurry	1	630	90	6 carb, 1 fat

Subway

Food	Size	Calories	Carbohydrate (grams)	Exchanges
Club	1 6-inch	312	46	3 carb, 2 lean meat
Roast Beef	1 6-inch	303	45	3 carb, 2 lean meat
Turkey Breast	1 6-inch	289	46	3 carb, 1 medium-fat meat
Meatball	1 6-inch	419	51	3½ carb, 1 medium-fat meat, 2 fat
Chocolate Chip Cookie	1	234	33	2 carb, 2 fat

Taco Bell

Food	Size	Calories	Carbohydrate (grams)	Exchanges
Double Decker Taco	1	330	37	2½ carb, 1 medium-fat meat, 2 fat
Soft Taco	1	210	20	1 carb, 1 medium-fat meat, 1 fat
Big Beef Burrito	1	510	52	3½ carb, 2 medium-fat meat, 3 fat
Grilled Chicken Burrito	1	390	49	3 carb, 1 medium-fat meat, 2 fat
Baja Chicken Chalupa	1	400	28	2 carb, 2 medium-fat meat, 3 fat
Nachos	1	320	34	2 carb, 4 fat
Cheese Quesadilla	1	350	31	2 carb, 1 medium-fat meat, 3 fat

KFC

Food	Size	Calories	Carbohydrate (grams)	Exchanges
Breast, no skin	1	169	1	4 lean meat
Breast, Original Recipe	1	400	16	1 carb, 4 medium fat meat, 1 fat
Breast, Tasty Crispy	1	470	25	1½ carb, 4 medium-fat meat, 2 fat
Breast, Hot and Spicy	1	530	23	1½ carb, 4 medium-fat, 3 fat
Chicken Pot Pie	1	770	69	4½ carb, 2 medium-fat meat, 6 fat
Biscuit	1	180	20	2 carb, 1 fat
Macaroni & Cheese	1	180	21	1½ carb, 2 fat
Mashed Potatoes with Gravy	1	120	17	1 carb, 1 fat

Pizza Hut

Food	Size	Calories	Carbohydrate (grams)	Exchanges
Meatless Taco, Thin 'N Crispy	1 medium slice	230	27	2 carb, 2 fat
Veggie Lover's Thin 'N Crispy	1 medium slice	222	30	2 carb, 1 medium-fat meat, 1 fat
Italian Sausage, Thin 'N Crispy	1 medium slice	325	45	3 carb, 1 medium-fat meat, 3 fat
Italian Sausage, Hand-Toss	1 medium slice	363	44	3 carb, 1 medium-fat meat, 2 fat
Italian Sausage, Pan	1 medium slice	415	45	3 carb, 1 medium-fat meat, 3 fat
Hot Wings	4	210	4	3 medium-fat meat

Brown Bag (from home)

Food	Size	Calories	Carbohydrate (grams)	Exchanges
Sandwich: 2 oz lean meat, tomato slices, lettuce leaf, spicy mustard, 1 tablespoon low-fat mayonnaise	1 whole sandwich	305	30	2 carb, 2 lean meat, 1 fat
Fruit	1 serving	60	15	1 carb
Carrot sticks	½ cup	25	5	1 vegetable

Source: Nutrient information from Holzmeister, LA: *The Diabetes Carbohydrate and Fat Gram Guide.* American Diabetes Association, Alexandria, Virginia, and American Dietetic Association, Chicago, Illinois, 2000.

Ethnic Food Guide

I t's important to be able to enjoy a wide variety of foods with
your food plan. The following tables give the carbohydrate
amount and exchanges for a selection of ethnic foods—Chinese
American, Indian and Pakistani, Jewish, and Mexican American. For
information on foods not listed here, check food labels at the grocery stores, ask at restaurants or ask friends how a food is prepared,
read ethnic cookbooks for descriptions, ask your dietitian, and
check carbohydrate gram books.

In the column titled Exchanges, "carb" includes foods in the
starch, fruit, and milk groups. You can either count a food as a carbohydrate serving or as a serving from the specific food group.
These tables are adapted from the *Ethnic and Regional Food Practices
Series,* 1989–1996, of the American Dietetic Association and American Diabetes Association.

Chinese American

Food	Serving Size	Calories	Carbohydrate (grams)	Exchanges
Starch				
Cellophane or mung bean noodles, cooked	¾ cup	73	18	1 carb
Ginkgo seeds, canned	¾ cup	86	17	1 carb
Lotus root, ¼ in. thick, 2½ in. round, raw	10 slices	45	14	1 carb
Mung beans or green gram beans, cooked	⅓ cup	71	13	1 carb
Red beans, cooked	⅓ cup	61	11	1 carb
Rice congee or soup	¾ cup	69	15	1 carb
Rice vermicelli, or noodles, cooked	½ cup	99	13	1 carb
Taro, cooked	⅓ cup	62	15	1 carb
Carambola or star fruit, medium, raw	1½	63	15	1 carb
Chinese banana, dwarf, raw	1	72	18	1 carb
Fruit				
Guava, medium, raw	1½	69	16	1 carb
Kumquats, medium, raw	5	60	16	1 carb
Litchi or lychee, raw	10	60	16	1 carb
Litchi or lychee, canned, drained	½ cup	57	15	1 carb
Longan, raw	30	60	14	1 carb
Longan, canned, drained	¾ cup	68	14	1 carb
Mango, small raw	½	68	18	1 carb
Papaya, raw, 3½ in. round, 5⅛ in. high	½	59	15	1 carb
Persimmon, Japanese (soft type), raw	½	59	16	1 carb
Pummelo, raw	¾ cup	58	14	1 carb
Milk				
Soybean milk, unsweetened	1 cup	78	4	1 carb

Food	Serving Size	Calories	Carbohydrate (grams)	Exchanges
Vegetables				
Amaranth or Chinese spinach, cooked	½ cup	14	3	1 vegetable
Arrowheads, or fresh corms, large, raw	1	25	5	1 vegetable
Bamboo shoots, canned	½ cup	25	4	1 vegetable
Bittermelon or bitter gourd, raw	1 cup	28	7	1 vegetable
Choyote, raw	1 cup	32	7	1 vegetable
Chinese celery, raw	1 cup	26	7	1 vegetable
Chinese eggplant, white or purple, cooked	½ cup	20	5	1 vegetable
Chinese or black mushroom, dried	2 medium	22	0	1 vegetable
Hairy melon or hairy cucumber, raw	1 cup	22	5	1 vegetable
Leeks, cooked	½ cup	16	4	1 vegetable
Luffa, angled or smooth, raw	1 cup	30	7	1 vegetable
Mung bean sprouts, with seeds, raw	1 cup	32	6	1 vegetable
Mustard greens, cooked	½ cup	11	2	1 vegetable
Peapods or sugar peas, cooked	½ cup	34	6	1 vegetable
Soybean sprouts, with seed, cooked or raw	½ cup	45	4	1 vegetable
Straw mushrooms	½ cup	20	4	1 vegetable
Turnip, raw	1 cup	36	8	1 vegetable
Water chestnuts, canned	½ cup	38	9	1 vegetable
Water chestnuts, raw	4 whole	35	9	1 vegetable
Winter melon or wax gourd, raw	1 cup	17	4	1 vegetable
Yard-long beans, raw	1 cup	44	8	1 vegetable
Meat and Meat Substitutes				
Mock duck or wheat gluten, canned	½ cup	88	10	½ carb, 1 lean meat
Beef jerky	1 3½ in. × 1 in. piece, ½ oz	44	1	1 lean meat

(continued)

Chinese American *(continued)*

Food	Serving Size	Calories	Carbohydrate (grams)	Exchanges
Scallop, dried	1 large	44	1	1 lean meat
Shrimp, dried	1 Tbsp or 10 medium	40	2	1 lean meat
Soybeans, cooked	3 Tbsp	56	3	1 lean meat
Squid, raw	2 oz	52	2	1 lean meat
Tripe, beef, raw	2 oz	56	0	1 lean meat
Beef tongue	1 oz	81	0	1 medium-fat meat
Tofu or soybean curd	½ cup, 4 oz	94	2	1 medium-fat meat
Duck egg, salted	1	137	0	1 medium-fat meat
Duck egg, preserved limed	1	114	3	1 medium-fat meat
Chinese sausage	2 oz	199	4	1 high-fat meat, 1 fat

Fat

Food	Serving Size	Calories	Carbohydrate (grams)	Exchanges
Coconut milk	1 Tbsp	35	1	1 fat
Sesame paste	1½ tsp	48	2	1 fat
Seasame seeds, whole, dried	1 Tbsp	52	5	1 fat

Free Food

Food	Serving Size	Calories	Carbohydrate (grams)	Exchanges
Amaranth or Chinese spinach, raw	1 cup	7	2	Free
Bok choy, raw	1 cup	10	2	Free
Chili pepper, raw	1	18	4	Free
Chinese or Peking cabbage, raw	1 cup	12	3	Free
Choy sum or Chinese flowering cabbage, raw	1 cup	9	2	Free
Coriander, raw	½ cup	2	0	Free
Garland chrysanthemum, raw	1 cup	4	1	Free
Ginger root, raw	¼ cup	17	4	Free

Food	Serving Size	Calories	Carbohydrate (grams)	Exchanges
Mustard greens, salted and soured	2 Tbsp	14	4	Free
Oriental radish or daikon, raw	1 cup	16	2	Free
Watercress, raw	1 cup	4	4	Free

Indian and Pakistani

Food	Serving Size	Calories	Carbohydrate (grams)	Exchanges
Starch				
Aviyal	½ cup	81	14	1 carb
Idli, plain, steamed	3 in. round	70	12	1 carb
Naan	¼ of 8 × 2 in.	75	13	1 carb
Phulka/Chappathi/Sookhi roti	6 in. round	68	15	1 carb
Plantain, green, cooked	⅓ cup	60	16	1 carb
Rice, regular, basmati, or jasmine, cooked	⅓ cup	69	15	1 carb
Sambar	½ cup	88	16	1 carb
Dhansak	½ cup	104	15	1 carb, 1 fat
Dhakla, khaman	1 in, square	104	12	1 carb, 1 fat
Matki usal	½ cup	104	10	1 carb, 1 fat
Pesrattu	9 in. round	127	14	1 carb, 1 fat
Poha	½ cup	140	18	1 carb, 1 fat
Puri	5 in. round	128	16	1 carb, 1 fat
Tomato dhal	½ cup	132	18	1 carb, 1 very lean meat
Toor dhal (red gram/split pigeon pea), plain, cooked	½ cup	103	20	1 carb, 1 very lean meat

(continued)

Indian and Pakistani *(continued)*

Food	Serving Size	Calories	Carbohydrate (grams)	Exchanges
Mung dhal (green gram), plain, cooked	½ cup	107	19	1 carb, 1 very lean meat
Garbanzo and most other beans, plain, cooked	½ cup	134	13	1 carb, 1 very lean meat
Fruit				
Mango, small, raw	½ cup	68	18	1 carb
Guava, medium, raw	1½	61	14	1 carb
Milk				
Lassi (blended nonfat yogurt)	1 cup	90	13	1 carb
Paneer	1 ounce	103	12	1 carb
Vegetables				
Brinjal (eggplant), plain, cookded	½ cup	13	3	1 vegetable
Cucumber raita	½ cup	21	3	1 vegetable
Karela (bittermelon/gourd), plain, cooked	½ cup	12	3	1 vegetable
Lady's fingers (okra), plain, cooked	½ cup	34	8	1 vegetable
Mung bean sprouts, cooked	½ cup	12	3	1 vegetable
Meat and Meat Substitutes				
Chicken, baked, spiced (no skin)	1 oz	54	0	1 lean meat
Chicken tikka (no skin)	3 1-in. pieces	54	0	1 lean meat
Chicken, tandoori (no skin)	1 ounce	75	2	1 lean meat
Fat				
Coconut, shredded	3 Tbsp	53	2	1 fat
Ghee (clarified butter)	1 tsp	45	0	1 fat
Oil (sesame, coconut, mustard, peanut)	1 tsp	40	0	1 fat

Free Foods

Chai massala (spice tea)	½ cup	14	3	Free
Coriander, fresh	½ cup	2	0	Free
Ginger, fresh and dried	¼ cup	17	4	Free
Jheera pani	½ cup	16	3	Free
Rasam	1 cup	22	2	Free

Jewish

Food	Serving Size	Calories	Carbohydrate (grams)	Exchanges
Starch				
Bulgur, cooked	½ cup	76	17	1 carb
Bulke	½ medium	76	14	1 carb
Farfel (dry)	½ cup	90	20	1 carb
Hallah	1 slice (1 oz)	85	14	1 carb
Kasha (cooked)	½ cup	91	20	1 carb
Kasha (raw)	2 Tbsp	71	15	1 carb
Lentils	⅓ cup	77	13	1 carb
Matzoh	¾ ounce	86	17	1 carb
Matzoh meal	2½ Tbsp	86	18	1 carb
Potato starch (flour)	2 Tbsp	79	18	1 carb
Pumpernickel bread	1 slice (1 oz)	69	15	1 carb
Rye bread	1 slice (1 oz)	68	15	1 carb
Split peas	⅓ cup	77	14	1 carb
Matzoh ball	3 balls (1½ oz)	134	17	1 carb, 1 fat
Potato pancake	½ pancake	119	13	1 carb, 1 fat
Vegetables				
Borscht (no sugar or sour cream)	½ cup	38	5	1 vegetable
Sorrel, cooked	½ cup	14	2	1 vegetable

(continued)

Jewish *(continued)*

Food	Serving Size	Calories	Carbohydrate (grams)	Exchanges
Meat and Meat Substitutes				
Flanken	1 oz	57	0	1 lean meat
Gefilte fish, broth	2 oz	48	4	1 lean meat
Herring (smoked, uncreamed)	1 oz	61	0	1 lean meat
Lox	1 oz	33	0	1 lean meat
Sardines (canned, drained)	2 medium	50	0	1 lean meat
Smelts	1 oz	35	0	1 lean meat
Beef tongue	1 oz	81	0	1 medium-fat meat
Brisket	1 oz	69	0	1 medium-fat meat
Chopped liver	¼ cup	75	3	1 medium-fat meat
Corned beef	1 oz	72	0	1 medium-fat meat
Sablefish, smoked	1 oz	73	0	1 medium-fat meat
Salmon (canned)	¼ cup	79	0	1 medium-fat meat
Pastrami	1 oz	99	1	1 high-fat meat
Fat				
Cream cheese	1 Tbsp	49	0	1 fat
Nondairy creamer (liquid)	2 Tbsp	40	3	1 fat
Nondairy creamer (powder)	4 tsp	44	4	1 fat
Schmaltz	1 tsp	31	0	1 fat
Sour cream	2 Tbsp	52	1	1 fat
Free Foods				
Horseradish	1 Tbsp	6	4	Free
Pickles, dill	1	7	1	Free

Mexican American

Food	Serving Size	Calories	Carbohydrate (grams)	Exchanges
Starch				
Bolillo (French roll), 4½–5 in. long	¼	87	17	1 carb
Frijoles cocidos (cooked beans)	⅓ cup	77	14	1 carb
Frijoles cocidos	1 cup	210	28	2 carb, 1 lean meat
Frijoles refritos (refried beans, no fat added)	⅓ cup	89	16	1 carb
Frijoles refritos (fat added)	⅓ cup	122	12	1 carb, 1 fat
Tortilla, corn	1, 7½ in. across	69	13	1 carb
Tortilla, flour	1, 7 in. across	118	22	1½ carb
Tortilla, flour	⅓ of 9 in. across	65	12	1 carb
Pan dulce (sweet bread)	1, 4½ in. across	384	61	4 carb, 1 fat
Fruit				
Mango	½ cup	68	17	1 carb
Papaya	1 cup	54	14	1 carb
Vegetables				
Chayote (squash), cooked	½ cup	19	4	1 vegetable
Jicama (yambean root), raw and cooked	½ cup	23	5	1 vegetable
Nopales (cactus), raw	½ cup	24	6	1 vegetable
Meat and Meat Substitutes				
Menudo (tripe soup)	½ cup	55	2	1 lean meat
Queso fresco (cheese made with skim milk)	¼ cup (2 oz)	80	2	1 medium-fat meat
Chorizo (Mexican sausage)	1 ounce	132	0	1 high-fat meat, 1 fat
Avocado	⅛ medium	40	2	1 fat

(continu

Mexican American *(continued)*

Food	Serving Size	Calories	Carbohydrate (grams)	Exchanges
Free Foods				
Jalapeno chilis, canned	½ cup	17	3	Free
Salsa de chile (chili/taco sauce)	2 Tbsp	13	3	Free
Verdolagas (purslane), cooked	½ cup	10	2	Free

APPENDIX G

Glycemic Index Guide

There are many factors that affect the blood glucose response to a meal. You can use the food experiment steps in the table on page 80 to help determine if a food has an influence on your blood glucose results. Also refer to chapter 10 for a description of the glycemic index.

GLYCEMIC INDEX (GI) RANGES

For convenience, foods can be divided into three broad categories: low-glycemic foods (with index values less than 55), intermediate-glycemic foods (with values between 55 and 70), and high-glycemic foods (with values over 70). Here are some examples of which foods fit into which categories.

Glycemic Food	Amount	Index	Carbohydrate (grams)
Cereal			
All-bran with extra fiber	½ cup	51	22
Intermediate GI: Frosted Flakes	1 oz	55	28
High GI: Corn Chex	1 oz	83	26
Grapenuts	¼ cup	67	27
Life	¾ cup	66	25
Oatmeal, old-fashioned	1 cup	49	26
Special K	1 cup	54	22
Total	¾ cup	76	24

(continued)

Food	Amount	Glycemic Index	Carbohydrate (grams)
Bread			
Pumpernickel, whole grain	1 slice	51	15
Rye	1 slice	65	15
White	1 slice	70	12
Crackers			
Barley, cooked	½ cup	25	22
Rice cakes, plain	3 cakes	82	23
Soda crackers, saltine	8 crackers	74	17
Stoned wheat thins	3 crackers	67	15
Water crackers	3 large	78	18
Pretzels	1 ounce	83	22
Pasta			
Fettuccine, cooked	1 cup	32	57
Linguine, thin, cooked	1 cup	55	56
Macaroni, cooked	1 cup	45	52
Macaroni and cheese dinner	1 cup	64	48
Dried Beans and Starchy Vegetables			
Baked beans	½ cup	48	24
Black beans, boiled	¾ cup	30	31
Chickpeas (garbanzo beans), boiled	½ cup	33	23
Corn, canned	½ cup	55	15
Kidney beans, red, canned	½ cup	52	19
Lentils, green or brown, boiled	½ cup	30	16
Potatoes, instant mashed	½ cup	86	14
Sweet potato, peeled, boiled, mashed	½ cup	54	20
Potato, white-skinned, mashed	½ cup	70	20
Potato, white-skinned, unpeeled, baked	1 medium	85	30
Fruit			
Apple, fresh	1 medium	38	18
Apple juice, unsweetened	1 cup	40	29
Banana, fresh	1 medium	57	32
Cantaloupe, fresh	¼ small	65	16

Food	Amount	Glycemic Index	Carbohydrate (grams)
Dates, dried	5	103	27
Fruit cocktail, canned in juice	½ cup	55	15
Orange, fresh	1 medium	44	10
Papaya	½ medium	58	14
Raisins	¼ cup	64	28
Watermelon	1 cup	72	8
Grains			
Couscous, cooked	½ cup	65	21
Rice, brown, cooked	1 cup	55	37
Rice, instant, cooked	1 cup	87	37
Rice, white, long grain, cooked	1 cup	56	42
Rice, white, short grain, cooked	1 cup	72	42
Candy and Desserts			
Angel food cake	¹⁄₁₂ cake	67	17
Banana bread	1 slice	47	46
Chocolate bar	1½ ounces	49	26
Doughnut with cinnamon and sugar	1 (1.6 oz)	76	29
Glucose tablets	2½ tablets	102	10
Jelly beans	10 large	80	26
M&M's chocolate candies, peanut	½-oz package	33	30
Mars Almond Bar	⅛ oz	65	31
Oatmeal cookie	1	55	12
Skittles, fruit bite-size candy	2.3-oz package	70	59
Sucrose (table sugar)	1 tsp	65	4
Vanilla wafers	7	77	21

Source: Brand-Miller, J; Wolever, TMS; Colagiuri, S; Foster-Powell, K; *The Glucose Revolution.* Marlowe & Company, New York, 1999. Adapted with permission by the *American Journal of Clinical Nutrition.* © American Journal of Clinical Nutrition. American Society for Clinical Nutrition.

Index

Numbers in *italics* indicate charts or tables.

270 INDEX

Healthy Food Choices, 186
heart disease, 122, 155, 156–58, 208
hemoglobin A1C tests, 28. See also A1C tests
Hendley, J., 57
herbal supplements, 164
high-protein diets, 146
holidays, food plans for, 55–56
hormone fluctuations, blood glucose and, 76–77
How Much Fiber to Eat Each Day, 133
How to Experiment with Food to Determine Its Impact on Your Blood Glucose, 80
How to Increase Fiber Intake, 135
How to Increase Whole-Grain Intake, 137
Humalog (lispro), 17
hypoglycemia, 104. See also blood glucose, low
hypoglycemia unawareness, 109
hydrogenated fats, 153
hypertension, 148, 164–66

infections, 75–76
ingredients, staple, 52–53
ingredients lists, on food labels, 215–16
insulin, natural
  deficiency, 22
  fat and, 13
  food and, 13, 41
  glucose and, 13
  lack of, 13

protein and, 13
resistance, 22, 93
role of, 13
insulin shock, 104. See also blood glucose, low
insulin treatment
  action times, 17
  activity and, 84, 85, 87
  adjusting, 177–82
  background, 17
  blood glucose and, 16, 20, 73, 103, 112, 177–82
  bolus, 17
  carbohydrate counting and, 48, 177–82
  correction factors, 181, 182
  effects of, 17, 18–20
  1,500 and 1,800 Guides, 181–182
  food and, 16, 178–82
  gastroparesis and, 78
  for gestational diabetes, 25
  Insulin Action Times, 17
  Insulin Adjustment When Using Rapid-Acting Insulin and Correction Factor of 35, 182
  insulin-to-carbohydrate ratios, 177–82
  intermediate-acting, 16, 17, 18, 20
  long-acting, 17, 19
  low blood glucose and, 103, 112
  mealtime changes and, 197
  mixed, 16, 17, 18, 20–21
  plans, 15–21
  premixed, 16, 17, 20–21, 87
  pumps, 15, 16, 48, 73

sugars *(continued)*
  reducing amount of, 56–57, 58
  Sugar Descriptions You May
    See on Food Labels, *211*
  types of, 124–32
supplements, 163–64, *165*
surgery, blood glucose and, 80
sulfonylureas, 23, 84, 103, 112
sweeteners, low-calorie, 126–29

Take Control, 158
Ten Percent Guideline for weight
  loss, 95
10 to 20 Guidelines for weight
  loss, 95
thaumatin, 129
thiazolidinediones, 24
Tips for Estimating Food
  Portions, *204*
Tips for Reducing Sodium
  Intake, *166*
tocopherols, *163*
trans-unsaturated fats (trans
  fats), 152, *153*
travel, food plans during, 200
triglycerides, *155*
type 1 diabetes
  activity and, 89
  food plans and, 15
  incidence of, 15
  insulin plans for, 15–21
  ketones and, 159
  low blood glucose in, 103,
    109–111
  weight and, 91
type 2 diabetes
  children with, 21
  food plans for, 21, 22
  incidence of, 21

insulin (natural) and, 21, 22
insulin treatment for, 22
low blood glucose in, 103
medications for, 22, 23–24
progression of, 22
as risk factor, 21
weight and, 21, 90, 91

ultralente insulin, 17
unsaturated fats, 152–53
USDA Dietary Guidelines, *39*

valsalva maneuvers, 88
vanadium vanadate, *163*
vegetables, 136
vegetarian food plans, 147
vitamins
  A, *162*
  B_{12}, 147
  C, *163*
  D, *163*
  E, *163*
  My Nutritional Supplements,
    165
  niacin, *162*
  nicotinamide, *162*
  supplements, 163–64, *165*
  thiamin, *162*
  Vitamins, Minerals, and
    Diabetes, *161–63*
vomiting, 76

waist measurements, 92
weekend, changes in routines
  during, 198–99
weight, excess
  Body Mass Index and, 91–*92*
  determining, 91–93
  fat intake and, 149, 150

American Dietetic Association

With nearly 70,000 members, the Chicago-based American Dietetic Association is the nation's largest organization of food and nutrition professionals. ADA serves the public by promoting nutrition, health, and well-being.